THE SUMMER OF HER BALDNESS

CONSTRUCTS | The Constructs Series examines the ways in which the things we make change both our world and how we understand it. Authors in the series explore the constructive nature of the human artifact and the imagination and reflection that bring it into being.

SERIES EDITORS | H. Randolph Swearer
Robert Mugerauer
Vivian Sobchack

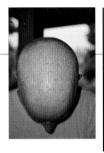

THE SUMMER OF

HER BALDNESS

a cancer improvisation

CATHERINE LORD

UNIVERSITY OF TEXAS PRESS, AUSTIN

The Summer of Her Baldness has been made possible, in very different and timely ways, by the Durfee Foundation and the Humanities Research Institute of the University of California. Portions of the book, printed here with the permission of the publishers, first appeared in *Art Journal* 61:1 (Spring 2002), published by the College Art Association, and in *GLQ: A Journal of Gay and Lesbian Studies* 9:1 (2003), published by Duke University Press. All photographs are by Catherine Lord.

First edition, 2004

Requests for permission to reproduce material from this work should be sent to Permissions, University of Texas Press, Box 7819, Austin, TX 78713-7819.

⊗ The paper used in this book meets the minimum requirements of ANSI/NISO Z 39.48-1992 (1997) (Permanence of Paper).

LIBRARY OF CONGRESS | Lord, Catherine, 1949–
CATALOGING-IN-   The summer of her baldness : a cancer improvisation / Catherine Lord.
PUBLICATION   — 1st ed.
DATA   p.   cm. (Constructs series)
Includes bibliographical references and index.
ISBN 0-292-70256-6 (cloth : alk. paper)
ISBN 0-292-70257-4 (pbk. : alk. paper)
1. Lord, Catherine. 2. Cancer in women. 3. Breast—Cancer—Biography.
4. Cancer—Patients—Biography. 5. Lesbian feminism. I. Title.
II. Series.
RC281.W65L67 2004
362.196'99449'0092—dc22   2003021616

TO KIM

AND

TO THE FRIENDS OF CATHERINE LORD'S RIGHT BREAST

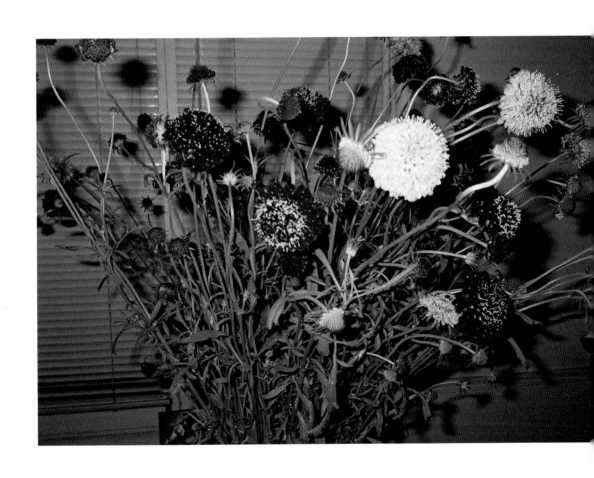

IN A MESSAGE DATED
6/1/01 CBLORD@UCI.EDU
WRITES TO UNDISCLOSED
RECIPIENTS:

SUBJECT: LOOKING BACKWARD
(CONFESSIONS OF HER BALDNESS)

On my computer, the name of this list serv, Her Baldness's own privately
maintained and preciously guarded list serv, is FOCL'SRB. It started
small—just the people I could squeeze into the phrase "friends and family." Her Baldness added to the list from time to time, in return for acts of
kindness that happened as the news of my breast cancer traveled—a call,
a postcard, a book propped by her front door, an email. Her Baldness also
subtracted. She got mad at people for not being there, or not being there
as much as she wanted, or not giving her feedback, much as she loathed
the word, or, conversely, giving her feedback, regurgitating what she didn't
want to see and telling her what she never wanted to hear about. Some
people restored themselves to her good graces. Some people were de-
leted forever. Occasionally, when Her Baldness put things in her missives that might have embarrassed her in front of certain people, she de-
leted those people until she had stopped talking about them and the
coast was clear. Her Baldness had her petty moments. She was manipula-
tive and she could be vindictive. She whined. Not only had she caught
cancer but she had contracted the two most common symptoms of cancer: Unwanted Aloneness and Loss of Control. Instead of being angry at
her cancer, or the idea of cancer, or evolution, or the medical profession,
or industrial polluters, or state misogyny, or advanced capitalism, she got
mad at people she knew. It's easier to get mad at people than it is to get
mad at cancer, and easier still to get mad at them by committing acts of
mingy bureaucracy, even if you yourself have invented the entire feeble
apparatus in a technologically amplified moment of rage and terror.

Her Baldness made up this list to put the telling in her voice, to warn
people to stay away from pity, to be remembered because she thought

she might die. She made up this list so that she could be strong and proud and brave and full of energy and motion in the middle of the desolation that is cyberspace, even if she hated how she looked and it took pretty much all she had sometimes to get down the stairs to the computer in her studio and stay there. She made up this list because people are not perfect. They give what they can. Sometimes they cannot afford much, and in times of crisis, even when people are lavish it does not feel like enough. Her Baldness figured that her miserable bald wobbly pale being could not expect to have sympathy pour in like water from the tap. She made up this list in order to have a place in which to write. She made up this list to create the people for whom she wanted to write. She made up this list because she needed an audience in order to stay alive. She plucked an audience out of thin air. Having done so, she played it shamelessly. She sang for her supper. She danced for her dinner. She stripped for sympathy. She posted her fear. She got off on the fact that all sorts of people were on the list and that none of the undisclosed recipients knew for certain the identity of any of the other undisclosed recipients. The highest compliment she received was archival in nature: "I save all your emails. I have numbered them." The second highest compliment she received was larcenous in nature: the (generally unauthorized) gesture of forwarding her emails to other people.

If I had accepted the prescription offered when my oncologist informed me that my insurance would cover chemo-induced alopecia, I would have gotten a piece of paper entitling me to a free cranial prosthesis, otherwise known as a wig, and Her Baldness would never have had to be invented. Her Baldness was another approach to the design of prosthetic devices, an honorific fabricated to point to the fact of mortality while at the same time waving at the colors of the sunset, a strategy designed to flaunt and to conceal. Her Baldness was a contradiction in terms, a loudmouth and a smokescreen, an avatar and a mask.

We had, Her Baldness and I, a conflicted relationship. At all times conscious of each other's intent and each other's strategy, we couldn't take our eyes off each other, so sometimes we didn't see the love we thought was missing when it was coming straight at us. We covered for each other. We used each other. We had no room for other people, even though we thought that pulling other people into our world was the point of the game. We had our roles, Her Baldness and I. Doubtless those roles had something to do with gender, among other possibilities, but it is not clear, even in retrospect, now that Her Baldness is in a state of hibernation, whether the man of the house caught cancer or the femme between the sheets. Whatever Her Baldness and I were doing, we switched off.

Her Baldness talked big, and Her Baldness talked a lot. Her other half, regrettably, was by no means bald and proud and loud. I myself never managed to go out of the house without a hat when I believed I was bald, though I did so when my hair was still so short that other people congratulated me on my courage for showing myself bald, thus making me feel even worse about my incurable shame and transparent cowardice. Her Baldness, on the other hand, though she spouted a good line, had places she would not go. She also had times, particularly when she was muddling her way through the minefield of getting well, that she could not pull herself out of her depression and write. Neither could I. Thus, there are holes in our collaboration. Huge holes. We are not holding out on you. Also, we contradicted ourselves and occasionally we lost our sense of irony. We didn't say thank you with much grace and sometimes we forgot altogether.

Some of you have asked how Her Baldness got started. What you are fishing for is not more information about the day my hair lost the battle and Her Baldness launched herself into the void like Yves Klein (who, after all, faked the photograph) or Thelma and Louise (who couldn't be allowed to live in America) or the postqueer hacker cyber assassin I wish I were (though that woman is younger, hasn't caught cancer yet, and has more energy than I do). You want to know about the moment when the woman who became Her Baldness in what she now prefers to describe as an involuntary performance piece learned that her life had changed. But in this narrative as in all others, it is a distraction and an impediment to think about a single moment of origin. It suggests something that could be repaired or rethought or restrung. You cannot find one single moment, however, when soft innocent tissue went wrong and turned into a monster that will grow unchecked until it bleeds its host to death. It is not a question of where you were when Kennedy was shot, if you are my age, but of considering where you were when Jackie died and remembering why.

There are, nonetheless, moments that are part of the story. It is both hard and unnecessary to choose between them. I shuffle them to emphasize that there is no hierarchy.

There was the day the gynecologist said she wasn't worried because the lump was mobile and she was sure it was just a cyst, so much so that she had to restrain herself from draining it on the spot. I asked her recently whether she was lying to me to give me a better week before the mammogram could be scheduled. No, she said, with some indignation, no, absolutely not. I don't entirely believe her.

There was the mammogram. Three retakes by Carlaloyce, who didn't know how she happened into her job, she never wanted to have a job that caused so many people discomfort with all the squishing and poking, but there it is, life is funny, she'd lost several members of her family to breast cancer and she needed to do this. The trouble is, Carlaloyce said, people get so mad at me when something comes out wrong. They yell and yell, but it's not my fault. That was another moment.

There was Natasha in ultrasound. Natasha was not chatty. Natasha called in the radiologist. They used a lot of blue goo. What's up? I asked. Don't talk to me right now, he said. I need to concentrate. That was another moment.

It took an entire box of giant medical kleenex to get the goo off. I felt like a porn movie extra. I got dressed and wandered the hallway. (Wrong. Women are supposed to stay in their cubicles until released by the proper authorities.) I bumped into the radiologist by accident. We need to talk, he said. The architect had apparently forgotten to design a room in which to deliver bad news, so the radiologist borrowed an office and moved someone's lunch off the desk chair. All the lumps are cysts but one and that lump, at twelve o'clock on your right breast, look here on the film, you can see, is a solid mass of one and a half centimeters. You need to get it biopsied. I advise you to take care of it immediately. That's another perfectly good moment.

There was the morning in April, sitting in the bathtub, when I soaped my breasts and my hand slid over a hardness that hadn't been there before. Another one.

There was the news of the biopsy report. Friday, May 26, 2000, on the 710 north, at about 4:30 in the afternoon, driving home to Los Angeles with my friend Annie after a long day teaching. Memorial Day weekend. I knew I couldn't wait for the results until Tuesday. I had called the surgeon's office at least four times. When I got through to Marcie the office manager she said the lump was suspicious. Do you want to talk to the surgeon? YES. So she patched me through to Dr. Phillips, presumably driving to a better location in a better car on a better freeway. It's true that the lab report doesn't use the word malignant, he said, they never do, but when they say suspicious it's 99% sure it's cancer. You can get another opinion, but this is a non-controversial course of action and I would advise you to schedule a lumpectomy and a sentinel node biopsy as soon as possible.

A footnote. When Her Baldness was a girl, growing up in the Caribbean on the island of Dominica, she didn't go to school at the usual age. Due to the combination of her resourcefulness and the extreme dysfunction of her family, no one noticed until she arrived in the classroom of a boarding school at the age of nine that she was severely nearsighted. When she got her first pair of glasses, she was astonished to learn that you could from a distance see the leaves she knew to be upon the trees and the waves she knew to make up the sea and the clouds she knew brought the rain she felt upon her skin. Until that moment, she believed that the rest of the world had either more memory or more imagination than she did, so that when, for example, they said, look over there at the hill to see the flowers on the tulip tree or look at the white caps out there by Scott's Head or look at the clouds coming in over Trois Pitons they had themselves walked to the tulip tree and returned to discuss among themselves what they remembered, or had gotten up early in the morning to take a boat to Scott's Head, or had agreed among themselves to speak about the wetness they felt on their skins by discussing things that were invisible in the blue above her head. She had misunderstood everything, especially the lightness of memory and the weight of voice. These would be lessons that she would have to learn over and over again.

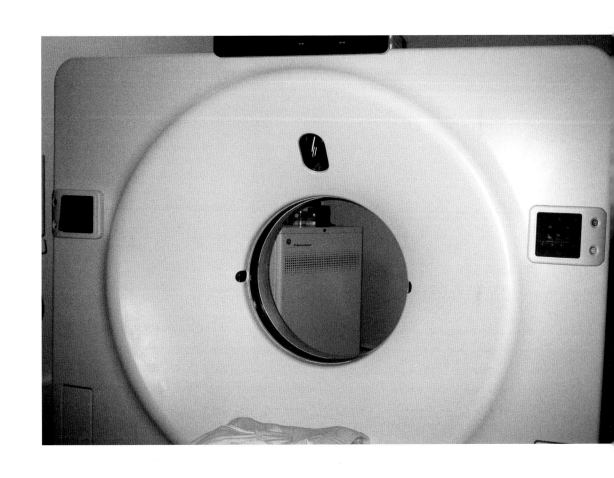

MAY/JUNE | 2000

My little sister calls from Florida. I'd rather spend the money it would take celebrating my fiftieth birthday coming to LA when you need me.

Mitchell calls. Do you have ANY idea how much I love you?

Dear friends and family:

That's as far as I get. You need to take care of yourself, not them, says the shrink. Don't worry about telling people yet.

Connie calls. She has been through it, with Jennifer and with her mother. Stock up on ginger tea, buy pot, get a wig. Dreads, we decide, because they are egregiously inappropriate, because I have always wanted them, and because why not? Buy a cordless doorbell. You don't always want people in your bedroom when you're feeling sick.

Junior calls. The twins wail in the background. What about a screening of the rough cut in a couple of weeks? We could invite Yvonne and Deb and Pattie and whoever. I tell her. She struggles. Will you be well enough to come to the screening? Later, I say. I can't decide right now.

Peggy calls from New York. She's a surgeon. Cancer is her thing. I didn't ask Dr. Phillips this morning in the hospital after surgery about my chances, but I ask Peggy. Now that you have at least one positive node, between 70 and 95%, she says. But there are different kinds of cancer. I can't say without the full pathology report because you don't know what kind it is and I don't know how many nodes are positive. Chemo will take three to six months. Radiation will be another six to eight weeks. In between you get a break.

My mother calls. I'm sorry. When you called this morning from the hospital I had lunch guests and I couldn't talk. She IS really sorry, that's the thing.

My department chair calls. We had a meeting. Where the hell were you? Oh NO, not you. He turns to the subject of new buildings. You have an enormous community, he says by way of farewell. I weep. I weep at moments of kindness. Tears are, as a shrink I once had remarked, only water. Logistically, however, it is difficult to speak and bawl at the same time. And the habit is embarrassing.

Dear friends and family:

Welcome to the epidemic.

I've just learned that I have breast cancer. I've had a lump removed, and I'll begin chemo in a few weeks. Then I'll probably need radiation. I know that some of you have been through this and much more. I hope you'll have advice, come visit on the good weeks that people keep assuring me will exist, and keep me posted about hot books, bad jokes and excellent gossip.

THURSDAY | JUNE 1, 2000

Did I think I would send that email?

My mother calls again, her anxiety welling and spilling. What about Linda's fiftieth? Will you be able to come to Iowa in July? My mother had a mammogram the same day I did. Hers was fine. Her mother had breast cancer.

I want to learn how to kayak. I want to write my book on Dominica. I want to retire and live with my love in a farmhouse in the country. I want to get a dog and swim in a swimming hole and eat corn and tomatoes. I want to go to New York in a few weeks. I want to be at my little sister's birthday party. I do not want to be a woman who is her breast cancer. I do not want to wear a pink ribbon and go on walks in crowds. I do not want people to practice the past tense. She was just pulling it together. She was in such good shape. She used to be so INTENSE but she'd mellowed. She was turning into a great person. I do not want to be stared at or whispered about. I want to be the person I never got around to being.

I grasp at straws. Deena's friend Betty had 53 positive nodes. That was twenty years ago, and Betty is going strong. Betty is my thickest straw. I watch people select their straws. As they recite the names of the survivors they know, I see them deleting from the list the names of the women who didn't make it. Here are the straws. Deborah and Yvonne and Sharon and Ellen and Annetta and Sean and Andrea and Ruth are just fine. Also Lizzie. Christine Tamblyn died, so did Kathy Acker, so did Jodi Carson, and so did Linda of Paul and Linda, and so did Hannah Wilke, but that was another kind, and so did Doug Heubler, but that was another kind still, and so did Catherine Hopkins, who wouldn't let go of my hand until I promised to take care of Kim forever. She died a few days after I made the promise.

Kim is scared. Kim is tender. Kim is terrified. When she doesn't think I'm watching, she falls apart. When I say her name she pulls her molecules together by an act of will and sits up straight. Let her be a rock for now, says the shrink.

Given the circumstances, is it appropriate to write notes about the cultivation of limes in Dominica in the nineteenth century? Am I insane to reduce my professional interests to an obsession about a small, poor, insignificant piece of rock in the Caribbean just because I happen to have been born there?

Flowers arrive from my mother. Get well soon. Love, Betty.

FRIDAY | JUNE 2, 2000

Dr. Phillips sails into the exam room. Only one lymph node is involved. There are studies that say one to three positive nodes mean the same survival rate as no nodes. Will I live? I ask him. You cannot imagine what it is like to find lines from a soap opera coming out of your mouth. YES, he says. Can I call you Ed? Yes.

A long time ago, Ed used to print for Ansel Adams. Perhaps the zone system made him fastidious. He didn't put a drain in under my arm and he saved the nerve, making this the one and only time in my entire life that I have benefited in any way whatsoever from Ansel Adams' theory of photography. You will be hairless, says Ed. Head, arms, legs, pubic hair, eyebrows. Eyelashes are the last to go. The standard chemo is three months. If the oncologist recommends Taxol as well, that will add another three months. Six to nine months is about right. Kim tells me afterwards that he came to her in the hospital waiting room, while I was recovering from the surgery, to tell her that the news was bad because he thought that nodes other than the sentinel node might be positive, and because he knew that I would have to have chemo.

Daniel calls. Omigod, he says, many times. OMIGOD. Do you have the best doctors?

Annie calls to be funny about wigs. I can't get there with her, and I am mad at her for being trivial.

Little is the best there is. Observe your mean places and let them go, the Buddhists would say.

OK, version 2.

Friends and family isn't the right way to begin, so dear people that, in one way or another, I love and/or care about and/or work with, here's a story. About two and a half weeks ago, my gynecologist said that the lumps I'd come to see her about were cysts. Since then, it's been a mammogram, and a needle biopsy (it doesn't feel like a new potato, so I'm optimistic, said the surgeon), and a lumpectomy and dissection of the lymph nodes and an overnight at Cedars (welcome to the world of bodily fluids the color of bad product shots for tropical cuisine). I have breast cancer. Details still coming in, doctors of various sorts still to be seen, but it looks pretty good for the long run, even though I will need chemo this summer to kill any errant cancer cells in my bloodstream and then radiation to the area of the original tumor. It will take somewhere between six and nine months.

I know some of you have been through this and much more. I hope you'll have advice (all kinds accepted, from the practical to the metaphysical). I hope you'll visit on the good weeks that people keep assuring me will be there, keep me posted about hot books, bad jokes, cool wigs and excellent gossip, and remind me when I need it which I doubtless will that this isn't the end of anything but the beginning of a process. I am no saint, so let me also say that it is a drag, did I say a fucking dismal nauseating drag and of course totally unfair. Nonetheless, I'm convinced that pleasures will be had in this sudden slowdown: writing that I am in the middle of writing, sweet moments with the world's greatest girlfriend, a lot of old movies, and cultivating friendships (which is why I am sending this to all of you, because I feel like I've had so little time to BE a friend and because I need to stay involved in things that matter to me intellectually and creatively and politically).

P.S. I don't plan on checking out of this planet anytime soon.

Cancer spam. To come out in the equivalent of a form letter seems to me entirely obscene.

SATURDAY | JUNE 3, 2000

Chloe wakes us in the middle of the night by sitting on my head and purring. I cannot get back to sleep. My restlessness wakes Kim. Kim heads for the sun porch. It occurs to me that because I disturb Kim's sleep, one of us will have to move out. Kim stumbles back to our bed crumpled and weeping for the first time since the nightmare began and I hold her tight in both arms, the bad one too. Her big beautiful face flushes and rumples and she wails herself to sleep. When we walk around the Silver Lake reservoir in the morning, there are seven or eight great blue heron nests, complete with spikey hungry babies, up in the eucalyptus.

Susan Love's Breast Book *arrives.*

I send out individual emails. No form letter. Only the subject heading is the same: A BIT OF BAD NEWS.

SUNDAY | JUNE 4, 2000

IN A MESSAGE DATED 6/4/00 LORRGRAD WRITES: Don't worry, honey, you will get LOTS of e-mail from me and jokes via my friend Sur.

IN A MESSAGE DATED 6/4/00 I.DJOSE WRITES: I'm sure this will be tough but luckily you're tough too.

It is early, I tell my department chair. I will finish the quarter. When you tell my colleagues, as I hope you will, because I do not want it to be a secret, I would prefer the following spin: SHE HAS BOTH TITS AND SHE AIN'T DEAD.

I waffle about chemo. Peggy calls. The cancer is no longer confined to your breast. That's what it means to have positive lymph nodes. It's in your bloodstream. You have one chance to get it out. If it comes back, you're in trouble. You're not a wimp. Eighty-year-old women get through chemo. Over my dead body will you decline it.

I fish for nice emails. None.

MONDAY | JUNE 5, 2000

IN A MESSAGE DATED
6/5/00 DEBOBR WRITES:
Bad jokes? The smarmy lady from the prosthesis company who visits you in the hospital peddling her array of wares. But then, I guess you'll be spared this treat since you're delumping instead of debreasting. You may get the wig lady, though personally I'd opt for the shaved head and some bad-ass caps.

The best part—and I really mean this—is getting a glimpse of all that we miss of the intensity and richness of life, blindered as we are by the pettiness and myopia of how we actually manage (or don't manage) to live it. Priorities will become much clearer.

IN A MESSAGE DATED
6/5/00 JEANNIES WRITES:
I think that's healthy to take sharing the news slowly. it gives you time to adjust to it yourself.

Party at Nathalie B.'s. I am amusing about activities that are not in my immediate future: Ashtanga yoga and air travel. I say nothing to anyone who does not already know. A lot of women have trouble telling people because they fear the pity. That's what Peggy said.

I scream in the car on the way back home. FUCKING BREAST CANCER!!! My armpit feels soggy—wet and numb and burning all at once.

TUESDAY | JUNE 6, 2000

IN A MESSAGE DATED
6/6/00 VOLT WRITES:
I know you're not made of iron but close enough.

IN A MESSAGE DATED
6/6/00 LIDAAB WRITES:
I have been sitting here for a while trying to write something but it is difficult. I hope you will feel better. I have learned a great deal working with you and thanks for everything.

Of the twenty-nine lymph nodes they took from the yellow fatty tissue of my armpit, one is positive. My tumor consists of white gritty tissue 1.7 cm x 1.5 cm x 1 cm. The margins are clear. I am the oncologist's job now. No weights or aerobics, Ed says, just walking the fingers slowly up the wall. You will be bald, he adds, but you'll be OK. You're young and strong. Goodbye kiss. It's all covered for six months, whatever you need, says Marcie in his office who has already come out to Kim. I wish WE got domestic partners insurance here. Home exhausted, to Susan Love. I pitch the

Fredericks (registered TM) polyester mesh mammary support system, AKA the huge itchy hospital bra. Too bad, said Kim. You had a full rack there for a while.

Bill from shrink. Not even a note inside.

No eyebrow pencil. No lipstick. No wig. No cartoon. I will cut my hair short before it goes.

Jeannie calls to offer to cook a meal.

Kim to the doddery Chloe in the middle of the night: IF YOU DIE THIS SUMMER I'LL KILL YOU!

WEDNESDAY | JUNE 7, 2000

IN A MESSAGE DATED 6/7/00 CBLORD@UCI.EDU WRITES TO CATGUN:

could we do a postscript scene for the *Object Lessons* video that consists either of me getting my head shaved, or getting my hair cut really really short? what about a week from tomorrow? verdict is 3 months chemo, then about two months radiation.

Irvine today to finish classes. Tears well. It's their faces. Can they fight down their own fear of their own death? Can they just be there?

Linda calls, as she does daily. Betty wants to visit for a weekend. I discourage this, remembering how hard it was last summer with the two of them in this small house. Kim doesn't need to take care of two more people.

Susan R. calls. What do you need us to do? Her doctor gave her fifteen years, in 1990. Don't try to be superwoman. Watch out for the people who back away from you.

Kim to Houston tomorrow, back on Friday, Miami on Sunday, back on the Monday to catch the first chemo on Tuesday. I am terrified she will miss the plane. I am terrified of barfing alone. Ask more of friends, says Annie. It's a reminder that you live alone and you die alone.

THURSDAY | JUNE 8, 2000

Five a.m. wake up, like a bird with no choice once the light reaches a certain level. The armpit incision is more secure. It seems unlikely to rip open. The incision on my right breast has healed sufficiently to let me sleep face down. I am lost. Do I read novels? How many? Should I cleanse body and mind of stress? Or would my attitude actually improve if I tried to be superwoman? What exactly is the difference between stress and energy?

People don't know what to do with me. They're trying to decide whether, or how, or when, to expel me from the social body. I don't have cancer, I am their cancer. I am a problem, an intruder, something to be cut out. At the same time I am joining the secret club of those who know what it is to fight and win. Or not. My cancer gives other people a chance to change. Their decision.

Nothing left to lose. Remember, speculate, invent, get it down, make language fly, whirl in my own baldness. My world, my language, my mind. A new gender. Breeze on the bald scalp. No eyebrows. No eyelashes. When it rains the water will run straight down into my eyes.

FRIDAY | JUNE 9, 2000

IN A MESSAGE DATED
6/9/00 SHARHA WRITES:
i think you should get one of those really really cool short hair cuts where your hair is about $\frac{1}{4}$ inch long. i love when people have their hair that short, it is so streamlined and strong. everybody will be touching your head like you're their cat.

SATURDAY | JUNE 10, 2000

Made it through airports to New York. I walk down Madison Ave. on a cool clear day. Someone else has cancer, not me, someone else will do chemo, not me, someone else will lose her hair, someone else will vomit. Someone else will be stared at because she has no eyebrows.

I run into Rhona B. outside the New School. Tears, again. Joke, again: My odds are good enough to let me die in a car crash on the way to Irvine.

It's like coming out of the closet. You don't do it just once, and once you've done it you can never stop. It's an act to be repeated again and again in different contexts. Cancer is a disease I can't just have, or be—that would be far too humane—but an identity I must state, or choose not to state, at every encounter.

Kim flies to New York from Miami and takes me to an insanely expensive dinner. You wouldn't do this unless I had breast cancer, I tell her.

IN A MESSAGE DATED   Instructor Lord, We all heard about your condition. I will pray for you.
6/12/00 LLCHONG WRITES:

I make lists of bald men. I invite them to dinner. I imagine a collectivity in which I would feel unremarkable.

I have very short hair. I do not have a buzz cut. All I have is cancer.

IN A MESSAGE DATED   We are all so glad you will come to Dominica in November and stay
6/14/00 HONYCHURCHS   with us. Marica has told us a terrible rumour—FRIENDS is discontin-
WRITES: ued and the last bit of news is that Chandler has married Monica. Is
this true?

Gray, cold, and my arm will not straighten.

I happen upon Margaret M. in a white box in Chelsea. Ooooo, nice haircut she says. I come out. She talks about a friend who just had a mastectomy. You don't have tits anyway, she adds. It won't matter. I stick them both out. I'll have chemo this summer, I tell her, but I hear it's not so bad these days. We'll have you and Kim to lunch, she replies.

Hat spree at Canal Jeans. Exhaustion.

IN A MESSAGE DATED   Chandler proposed, last Friends I caught, and NO there is no talk of it
6/16/00 CBLORD@UCI.EDU   being discontinued. That said, I have a bit of bad news about me. I
WRITES TO HONYCHURCHS: have just been diagnosed with breast cancer, which, let me emphasize,
is early, and very treatable indeed, though it is an epidemic among
women that I know. It has meant a bit of surgery (nothing radical, just
the lump out, and, oddly, I'm not even dented) and next, starting this
Tuesday, three months of chemotherapy followed by about the same of
radiation. It also means, to my immense sadness and disappointment,
that I cannot come and stay with you in Dominica in November.

Christine T. wrote to all the people she knew asking them to tell her what they thought the future would be and to give her stories of courage. She was about to have a stem cell transplant. She knew she would die. I didn't. Her cancer was three years too far along when it was discovered: a misread mammogram and a bad HMO. I wrote her back to say I didn't feel I had much courage.

SATURDAY | JUNE 17, 2000

IN A MESSAGE DATED 6/17/00 CBLORD@UCI.EDU WRITES TO SHARHA: it's not $1/4$ inch, yet, or just on the sides and the back, and one thing i've learned is that it will never be long again (i know, never say never) but finally i have reconciled myself to grandfather's ears and my grandmother's forehead. you have no idea the miniscule quantity of shampoo it takes to lather the fuzz.

Home to Los Angeles. Kim and I go to the pharmacist to pick up the first round of anti-barf pills. I need four. The pharmacist gives me three. We owe you one, she says breezily. That's not acceptable, I reply. I'm having chemo on Tuesday and I need the full prescription, which I ordered a week ago precisely so that you could have sufficient time to fill it. After fluttering and muttering she produces the fourth pill, but then flatly refuses to input any refills on the computer. I go postal. You know what this medication is for!! You KNOW no one uses it only once!! You KNOW this is not a recreational drug!!!!!!!!

A soup of seeded cucumber in chicken broth with a lot of butter. I want details so thick I can't see through them.

SUNDAY | JUNE 18, 2000

Cathy O.'s goodbye party. I tell Matias. He tells me he tested positive two months ago. Kathy Acker refused chemo and radiation, he says, but she died with her eyes open. I'm intuitive, he says. I'm right about things. You're going to make it.

Deep River opening, Ken G. whispers his sympathy. He knows from Susan and Robbert. They told him not to tell anyone. I'm not ashamed, I protest. Tell people. His boyfriend hugs me: we lost my sister to breast cancer last year. Daniel, ever sweet, promises to make little photographs, Ulysses tried to call but didn't want to talk into a machine, Deirdre warm, Jennifer funny, Lida scared, Mark too, Mario tender, Cirilo real. My mother said the worst thing about chemo was that it made everything taste like steel. Cirilo's mother died. You have to fight, he tells me, clenching his little fists. Kim and I sit on the sidewalk outside the gallery. I rub her back. Cirilo rubs mine. We are utterly at ease.

The haircut makes me lighter. I have the head I have, and the ears and the neck and the forehead and the eyes. And the mind. It is what it is. Other people can see me and I can see them. Nothing blocks my vision except for my tears, which come when I feel warmth or shock or love or concern or other people's fears of their own death, and even so I mind the tears less and less. They well and fill and overflow and they pass. My skin feels thin, air touching it on one side, water on the other, the sadness inside liquid so that it pours from my eyes. Less pretense, less armor, less carapace. When people ask me why I didn't do this before they are talking about things other than the haircut. Your face shines out now, Mario remarked.

All of a sudden, people are only people, mortal, imperfect, fragile, ephemeral, obliged from time to time to suffer. The baldness of my summer. This is all there is, sitting on a sidewalk on a summer night with a bunch of artists trying to make themselves into a scene, people who know as little about connecting as I do.

MONDAY | JUNE 19, 2000

IN A MESSAGE DATED 6/19/00 DEBOBR WRITES: Playing the numbers along with you . . .

IN A MESSAGE DATED 6/19/00 DANGERMOUSE WRITES: fight back, like never before remember any thing you need 24/7 just call you are not alone

Annie called yesterday to say she can't keep me company after chemo on Tuesday because she forgot she had a shrink appointment and also she has errands but she can come late on Wednesday and also she might need us to feed her cats on Friday. This is the person I think of as my best friend in Los Angeles. In fairness, she is drowning: Her grandmother is dying, her mother had breast cancer this spring. But what does fairness have to do with it? Desolation burns my eyes. I remind myself to set my expectations low.

I'd be there the next day if you wanted me, Linda says. She is scared. Me too. The worst is the not knowing. How long will it take? What color is it? How much exactly will it sting? How many times will I get stuck in order for them to find a vein? What will it feel like to have liquid flowing in rather than liquid flowing out? How to imagine a substance that causes your hair to flee from its follicles being good for you?

If the oncologist explained any of these details, I don't remember a thing. I call his nurse. Four rounds of Adriamycin and Cytoxan. Take Kytril an hour before the first visit. For the other visits

don't take the Kytril until you come in, because if your blood count is too low they may delay the chemo. You should be done with chemo by the end of August, which means radiation can start mid-September, probably thirty to thirty-five treatments. You'll need to allow time to rest up for a few weeks, so don't count on going anywhere until after Thanksgiving.

Everything will make you tired.

I keep reworking my calendar.

TUESDAY | JUNE 20, 2000

One down. Lightheaded, a bit of a headache, don't much feel like eating. The chemo is not as bad as the squabble about Kim's driving on the way there. You drive like an old lady. Stop. Look. Drift. Only on the freeway are you butch. Nothing hurts exactly but it's unnerving to watch liquids dripping in: anti-barf medication, then red Adriamycin, then clear Cytoxan. I chat with Michelle the nurse. Do you see people change? Yes, they start living. The worst thing is to stay home and ruminate. Staying home and ruminating is what I do for a living, I reply. Well, she says, after a long pause, don't get stuck.

Dr. Van Scoy Mosher looks puzzled when I ask but says that cancer is a hard white thing, usually very hard. Beating this is a lot about attitude. Most women are cured by the surgery. Chemo and radiation are precautionary measures.

What happened to my tumor? It's somewhere in Cedars. No, you cannot photograph it.

Buh-bye, new potato.

WEDNESDAY | JUNE 21, 2000

Nath calls. We have stayed away from each other for fifteen years. I love you. Do you want me to come? Ne lache pas. Don't let go.

Ken M. wants a letter of recommendation. OK, I say. I don't come out. It's hard to tell the people who just want something out of you.

The voice mail at the benefits office is full. Still shaky, light-headed, tired, especially of the sight of books about cancer. I have become a food nazi. Organic absolutely everything, pure this, unadulterated that, no oil but olive oil, only olive oil from Italy and only olive oil from Italy certified organic. Brown rice. Miso. Seaweed. I don't know how to cook seaweed. Nothing to pollute the already polluted body.

IN A MESSAGE DATED 6/23/00 CBLORD@UCI.EDU WRITES TO UNDISCLOSED RECIPIENTS:

SUBJECT: ANSWERS TO MOST FREQUENTLY ASKED QUESTIONS

There are twelve kinds of breast cancer: infiltrating ductal, invasive lobular, medullary, mucinous, tubular, adenocystic, papillary, carcinosarcoma, Paget's disease, inflammatory, and in situ, either ductal or lobular. One in eight women will get one of them by the time she is eighty. A few years ago it was one in nine. Some people say it's now one in seven.

Yes I have Susan Love's *Breast Book*. What I can't imagine growing in me was there all along, probably for eleven years. The drawings make what I have, or had, look like a tomato thrown hard against a glass patio door. It's tissue gone wrong, interleaved with bad cells interleaved with good cells, bad cells leapfrogging through my bloodstream. It's called breast cancer, but it can show up anywhere: bones, liver, heart, lungs. My now vanished lump with irregular margins had about a billion and a half cancer cells which could even now be coursing through my veins.

Yes, I have read Susan Sontag. Cancer is the disease of the passionless and repressed, the disease seen as the sci fi disease, the steady, relentless march of the nonself under the skin of the self, the alien under the familiar, the visible. Cancer is fought with military metaphors: invasions, scans, counterattacks, and so forth. Freud, said Reich, was beautiful when he spoke, and so he got cancer of the mouth. This is the theory of the character producing the disease. Never mind the smell of cigar smoke.

Yes I have read Audre Lorde. One lump, unspecified size, no lymph nodes. She had a mastectomy but declined chemo and radiation on the grounds that they are carcinogenic. She died. She was obsessed with pain in ghost flesh. She wouldn't wear her prosthesis—lambswool in a pink pouch. Wrong color. The nurses told her that if she didn't wear her prosthesis it would be bad for the morale of other patients. I'm not as angry as she was, at least at the moment. It is conceivable that I might be in denial. Also, I have no need for a prosthesis, and even if I did it would be made in my color.

Yes, I have looked at videotapes on the subject. My yoga teacher gave me a tape of an interview with his colleague Susan, who had breast cancer four years ago. Here's an excerpt: Were there times you were just hanging on by a thread? Yes.

Yes I have found a support group. Kim and I went to an office park in Santa Monica. Cancer platitudes all over the walls. Hats hanging on a hat rack. Donations from the recovered? Sacrifices to the newly bald? Everyone friendly, everyone straight. We were welcomed by Betty in a pink sweatshirt, cursive type: PATIENTS FIGHTING FOR RECOVERY. Her legs are the size of my wrists. When I first got cancer, she said, twenty-three years ago, you went to bed with a bucket. The new anti-nausea drugs are wonderful. Be positive. Concentrate on recovering, if possible. This is the mantra, comma included. You can transform yourself from a victim to a victor. After joining a support group 88% feel less alone, 87% are happier, 82% gain hope, 75% improve their will to live, 72% improve their relationship with their loved one.

Yes, I have seen a nutritionist, Eve C., a fifty-six-year-old Australian with a bleached blond punk haircut who thirty years ago had two tumors in her thigh and then cervical cancer at which point she gave up on doctors and cleaned up her act. She doesn't approve of chemo and radiation. She tried to withhold judgment but she didn't try hard enough. I see you're a university professor, she remarked. Does that mean you don't have an open mind? I teach art, I countered and explain, apologetically, that I'm doing Western medicine because I know three people in more or less my situation who died because they didn't do chemo and radiation, not to mention the friend who is a cancer surgeon who told me that over her dead body would I not do chemo. Cancer might not be the reason your friends died, she replied.

We arrived at a truce: chemo will destroy my immune system, Eve will repair it. She placed small bottles of things around various parts of my body and asked me to resist her pushing my arm or my leg, as the case may be. According to her, my liver is in great shape and my kidneys aren't. I went off with admonitions (no chicken, no cow anything, no caffeine, no chocolate, no sugar) and various bottles of things involving elms and burdock and rhubarb and polarized water and selenium and calcium not to mention a copy of Eve's book, recipes in the back, leek and potato soup being especially fine in her mind, all to the tune of $184, payable when services are rendered. I pay. I'll dig burdock myself if it staves off mouth sores and painful shitting and thin skin in places I would rather not think about when the blood count drops. I suppose I needed someone to tell me that something of mine was in great shape. Why not pay $184 to have someone praise my liver?

Yes, Kim is supportive. She came home immediately when I called her from the traffic jam on the 710. She has promised to be there for every chemo. She has promised to be there period. Nonetheless, it is clear that every button we have between us will be pushed. For me, it's loss of control and the fear of isolation. These buttons were tender before cancer. For Kim it is the tendency to take care of others before she takes care of herself. She has a corporate job. She is gone all day and into the evening. She is a workaholic and this is not the time for her to get over it. Not only are the demands of her job real but she will need to get out of the invalid universe. She confessed a few days ago, when I had a moment of good cheer, that she didn't think she could stand nine months of my depression. I hadn't known I was depressed. I just thought I couldn't decide whether to put milk in my tea or water the garden. I am terrified that we will grow apart. What will be there for her? We have promised to make a little celebration for ourselves every weekend, emphasis on the little.

Yes, I've succumbed to stress. This is, after all, how I made my living for years. Suppressing anger is the professional obligation of deans or department chairs, both of which I have been, or for that matter university professors, which I am now. Plus, I've done wrong by my lovers, all of them. I refused to come home and take care of my mother when she had a hysterectomy. My sister didn't bother to ask me to visit when she had hers. I skipped my own father's funeral. I didn't get down with my friend Deborah's pain when her girlfriend had to deal with a bone marrow transplant. I couldn't write a story of courage for my dying colleague. I was too shy to stand up and say something at Ray's funeral. I was furious at Lizzie for catching breast cancer on top of her interminable depression. I wasn't sufficiently comforting when Lizzie's sister threw all the furniture out the window and shot herself in the head. We are all imperfect, every last one of us, but we would rather grasp this fact as an abstraction since the reality is in the details and we are the details. I came up way short when they were handing out compassion, because it was that or drown in other people's sorrows. That's one theory of catching cancer. There are various others, perhaps not so much ideas as an inventory: chlorides, pollutants, a melancholic disposition, constricting corsets, chewing the fat of dead animals, living under electrical wires, watching television, sitting in front of computer screens. Or the luck of the draw. Two grandmothers with breast cancer.

I don't send this.

SATURDAY | JUNE 24, 2000

Nothing is interesting. Kim does all the driving from Los Angeles to Point Reyes. This is our getaway, our ruse to get ourselves through.

SUNDAY | JUNE 25, 2000

Gray mornings. We treat ourselves to seventy dollars of gourmet cheese, then another thirty dollars, not to mention organic whatever we please. Money is an abstraction. Point Reyes is where Colette stayed with an insanely jealous girlfriend who set fire to the house they'd rented when they were leaving. That was thirty years ago.

You are feeling better, says my mother.

WEDNESDAY | JUNE 28, 2000

I eat enormous amounts. Strength. Seals and pelicans and elk and two black deer, a doe with her fawn hopping in stiff-legged delight at the sight of two lost lesbians who have hiked eight miles out of their way.

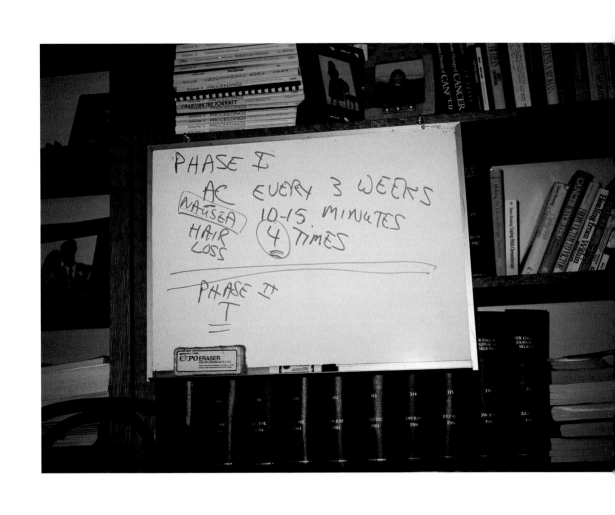

JULY | 2000

Back home to Silver Lake yesterday, on top of the world after ten days of vacation from cancer. Long walk and dinner with Annie. Yoga. Strands in the hair goo after my bath. Maybe it won't all fall out in chunks. Maybe I can watch without anticipating. Maybe.

Another breast book in the mail. Did I order it?

I weary of recipes for seaweed and greens and brown rice, the lists of what not to eat, the baths of baking soda and sea salt and hydrogen peroxide.

Shrink. Do you want to know how I feel? Mad, and sad that you have to go through this. You have so much to offer.

Still no word from the university benefits office about a medical leave.

TUESDAY | JULY 4, 2000

IN A MESSAGE DATED 7/4/00 CBLORD@UCI.EDU WRITES TO LDJOSE: my hair is beginning to fall out, just today. i miss you, and as i seek the company of the hairless (these reasons are not in order of importance), what about a movie?

Cold sores across my inner lip. Yoga anyway. Held my own. Hairs in the bath, straight and curly. OK. Three months. End of September. I have lost five pounds since May. I've got the padding.

WEDNESDAY | JULY 5, 2000

The distance widens. The significant events shrink to four chemos, one down, and seven weeks, maybe six, of radiation. I throw out bills for subscription renewals. I throw out movie schedules.

Ditto invitations. Do I want to go to the opening of an ex-student? No. The visual feminist meeting? No. I wobble when Kim goes back to work. I need friends but I save people up in case I might need them more later. I could easily pull out all my hair. Scratchy eyes. Scratchy eyelashes. Eddies of obsession.

The Perfect Storm at the Vista. I scan the calm blue sea for a speck. Kim and I are the only people in the audience stupid enough to think that George Clooney might live.

Yoga at home: four sun salutations, three standing poses, twists.

THURSDAY | JULY 6, 2000

IN A MESSAGE DATED 7/6/00 DEWDROP2U WRITES: Have you heard the new trend of dykes getting a star tattooed on their wrists, under where they usually wear their watches? . . . a reappropriation of lesbian factory workers during World War II. I'm thinking about getting one. Want to go together?

Nancy M. calls. I heard about it from Adam at the party for his new job. He didn't know what kind it was but he said he heard it was bad. Nobody else at the party knew either. How ARE you? Stacey Doran had it, didn't you hear about that, I thought you would have, and she didn't get any treatment besides surgery so she died in two years but you're DOING something, Catherine. You always were so PRACTICAL.

Metastatic art world gossip. I am being recategorized from invincible castrating lesbian bitch to has-been on her last legs. She used to be so tough. That's what they'll say. She must have gone downhill.

I want Nancy's attention but feel slimed because I am not in fact the focus. It's like sex with someone who doesn't give a shit whether you come.

Why do people tell you these things? asks Kim.

White blood count down from 4,900 two weeks ago to 2,900. I may or may not be able to have chemo next week. Meantime, no children, no groups where there might be sick people that I need to hug or air kiss. No gardening without gloves, no changing of kitty litter. Movies are OK. I have infiltrating ductal cancer, like 70% of the women who have breast cancer. Chest x-ray. Bone scan is under consideration. We can't tell how fast it is growing. It is her2neu positive and estrogen receptor negative. These are cause for concern.

Had I not felt a lump in the fall? Didn't you notice anything? asked the gynecologist. Would a few months have made any difference?

I am, this morning, strong enough to covet the last few days of hair.

FRIDAY | JULY 7, 2000

Kim's support group. Straight people, mostly men, partners of the terminal. Two hours of lives turned to shit. A woman hands out a clipping about groups for those who have lost pets.

Kim fails to meet her standards at work. She fails me by going to work. Even if I worry that my sister Linda will only want to shop for small things, I will ask her to come out from Florida for the next chemo. It will give something to both of us. I need to take the weight off Kim, who laments the fact that friends do not come through. I need to take care of myself.

You have to ask people directly, says the shrink. This is a special time for you. Do what you want. I ask Kim to teach me to dance. I make her a bouquet of yellows and whites and purples and greens at Gillyflowers, and tell the nice fag who asks how I am, more than once, because he asks more than once, what's going on. The flowers are for my girlfriend. Nobody has sent her flowers and she really needs people there for her. He has a friend who had a double mastectomy and is now getting her scars tattooed. You look OK, he says, staring at my breasts.

SATURDAY | JULY 8, 2000

Kim has a cold. She moves to the sun porch to sleep only to come back weeping in the middle of the night. We need to move to a bigger house so that I can have my own bedroom. I stand on the other side of the room and mime hugging her but I am pissed. How dare she run herself ragged? How can she get sick now? I don't want to wear a mask. I don't want life in a bubble.

Only one email this morning. My dean couldn't manage to tell her secretary to send me a sympathy card. My throat scratches. I can hardly move. Loss of control. Unwanted isolation. Textbook issues. Skin like paper. I stare at every cut and sore.

Shrink. Be bald. Take it as a badge of honor.

SUNDAY | JULY 9, 2000

I wake in the middle of the night gagging on the hair in my mouth.

IN A MESSAGE DATED
7/10/00 YSM WRITES:

Allan overheard someone at the Deep River opening mutter that you look more like Sigourney Weaver than ever with your short haircut.

IN A MESSAGE DATED
7/10/00 DEWDROP2U WRITES:

Me, Mary Ellen, Ann, and the kids are going to Coney Island tomorrow. Would you and Kim like to join?

IN A MESSAGE DATED
7/10/00 CBLORD@UCI.EDU
WRITES TO DEWDROP2U:

kim would love to go to coney island, and so would i, in a second, but we cannot make the morning plane.

IN A MESSAGE DATED
7/10/00 CBLORD@UCI.EDU
WRITES TO UNDISCLOSED
RECIPIENTS:

SUBJECT: OCCASIONAL MISSIVES FROM HER BALDNESS

I have been saying goodbye to my hair for a month and a half now, ever since I learned that the word chemo would be part of my future, though it is also true that for the same period of time I have suffered from an acute case of denial. Not my follicles. Not me. Even with Adriamycin/ Cytoxan, it takes a few chemos for some people to lose their hair.

The first act actually happened a month ago when I went to New York between surgery and chemo. Catherine Junior cut my hair. I have never in my entire life, except as an infant, had short hair, so the haircut was as much of a trauma, or I made it as much of a trauma, as the prospect of undergoing chemo. I choreographed for an atrocity. Mary Ellen would tape it. Kim would photograph it. The spectacle would run under the credits of the videotape on lesbian identities that Junior and I are making. I would go from long hair to buzz cut. Maybe I would smear lipstick on afterwards. It didn't turn out that way. Instead, I got a fabulous haircut in the company of three dykes who in one way or another love me. They talked me through. Why didn't you do this before? Why did you keep that terrible haircut for so long? If they measured you, you'd have an Aryan head. It wasn't clear whether the latter was supposed to make me feel better or worse, but it took me about five minutes to get with the program: outrageously mannish invert butchly LESBIAN haircut, the first one of my entire lesbian life.

I kept tugging on my hair after the first chemo, bragging to whoever would listen that it was still attached. LOOK. It's not falling out. Something in me had counted on another month or so among the haired. For the last week, however, it has been a different story. The errant cancer cells in my body have shriveled into dust, along with the cells that attach my hair to its follicles. Predictably and irritatingly in conjunction with the decline of the number of white blood cells in my body, my hair has become not MY hair but someone else's hair, as old and dry as hair from another century, a signifier that has detached itself from its time and drifted to my scalp where instead of sticking it came off on everything— bed pillows, sofa cushions, T-shirts, sweaters, car seat, kitchen sink, kitchen floor. In the bathtub, hairs straight and hairs curly.

I switched to wearing gray, not black. I began to brush my shoulders constantly. I began to rub my head more and more gingerly. Even though my scalp itched like hell, when I scratched it felt as if thousands of hair follicles were rebelling. Tingling is too mild to describe the sensation. It didn't hurt, but it felt wrong. My hair had no gloss, no curl, no spring. No moisture, no oil, no life. My hair was dead, a museum of female insecurity and lesbian codes. I stopped shampooing, figuring that if I left my hair alone perhaps it wouldn't make the effort to leave. I calculated the inevitable: maybe I could make it through my first support group, past my photo lab errand, past my movie date, past a MOCA visit. Friday night I woke up choking. When I turned on the light, my hair was all over the pillow. I was spitting my own hair out of my mouth. Even if the top of my head was still covered with hair, the hair had turned into dirt. I was my own horror film.

On Saturday, with David along for fashion advice, I went to Fred Segal's and got the perfect black cotton knit cap for an obscene amount of money. I needed to have a replacement before my hair and I parted ways. This is the only way I know to negotiate endings. I have never not been in a relationship.

On Sunday, Kim and I read *The New York Times*, heated leftover chicken soup for breakfast, and began. Better to stage the experience yourself than to have the experience stage you. Maybe if there were less hair, its own weight wouldn't drag it out of the follicles. Maybe a buzz cut would buy me a few days. We began with the top of my head, but when Kim let me look in the mirror, it was Marine Corps with dollar-sized shiny patches of bald. Mangy, said I. Auschwitz, said Kim.

We set the buzz shorter. Tiny black specks all over my T-shirt, the skin of my back and breasts, my legs and face, little pinpricks of history, jagged little reminders of the one and only month in my life with a great dyke haircut. I climbed into the bathtub, but when I shampooed it didn't stop. There were black specks on the pink of my palm every time I put my hand to my head. Finally, Kim knelt on the floor beside the tub and shaved me, talking me through it, rubbing my head and arms, saying again and again that I am beautiful, that my head is beautiful, that I am the most beautiful woman she's ever seen, that I am more beautiful than I used to be.

I climbed out of a tepid pond of scummy water, globs of hair floating on the surface, to look in the mirror. From the eyes down, I recognized the face about which I have always had such profound ambivalence and which has never been RIGHT or symmetrical or particularly striking much less, in honest fact, beautiful. The eyes are the midpoint of the head, which means that there is a lot of unfamiliar territory above, a lot of white skin that has never been touched by the sun, a lot of naked, bare, stripped, shorn, delicate, exposed, vulnerable and in fact the long inventory of words that teach us we are better masked in public, that masked in fact is our ticket into existence in public, our permission, that hair is something the strong strip from the weak, be they animals or wayward women or boot camp recruits. My skull felt thinner, as if it could crack wide open in a social setting, and the mirror in a middle-aged woman's bathroom is not a private place. It is irrevocably and inexorably a social setting.

I dug out my most ancient and disgusting second- or even perhaps third-hand thrift store pajamas, all the while thinking that in this the summer of my baldness I should be taking special care about appearances, and climbed into bed. It was three in the afternoon. Your hands are trembling, said Kim. The pate that I had just acquired was reflected in the screen of the television set.

When I woke, hours later, Kim had made dinner and cleaned up the worst tub ring in domestic history, an act of pure love, if you ask me. I am a bald woman. From the diagnosis on, this has been my worst fear. Dying? Way down on the list, way below amputation, which is in turn way below my second worst fear, that when bald I will discover rolls of fat on the back of my neck. There are none.

My first day out in the world as the star of my own horror movie was devoted to doctors—surgeon, shrink, and radiology lab. When you go to see professionals, they are not the only people that you see. There was the gas station attendant, the ten people in line at the photo lab where of course I ran into an art dealer (Catherine, what happened to all your hair?), the three people behind the counter at the drug store where I stopped to get ice packs and Tylenol for the next chemo, the parking lot attendant, the people in the elevator at Cedars, the guard who explained to me how to get to the ATM, the second parking lot attendant at the shrink's, the waiter at the Newsroom, where I decided to get lunch because it takes time to see doctors and you get hungry, the other forty or so well-heeled and well-haired customers in the restaurant, the other client in the shrink's waiting room, the third parking lot attendant, the ten people in the chest x-ray waiting room, the woman with the eight-inch scar down her neck and shoulder in the next booth, the x-ray technician, and the cashier.

This is my life. It has changed irrevocably but it is the only life I have. I need to make it a normal life.

I do not remove my hat in any of the doctors' offices, especially not the shrink's. It is a new relationship; we are not there. Of COURSE I'm displacing my anxiety about death, I say to her, but I'm not dead, I'm bald. Bald is all that's accessible.

By the time I get home, I ache to feel the afternoon breeze on my skull, though before I am safely inside I must explain to my inquisitive neighbor why I look different. He is speechless. His wife died of breast cancer last fall. You look very attractive, volunteers his new girlfriend. Mitchell, dear delicate fag with well-tended pate on the other side of the country, calls with advice: no sun for a week, it's much too sensitive, rub in lotion, wear big jewelry, try lipstick, what about African caps? Linda calls to say she has found restorative poses to open the part of the chest where the gland that controls the immune system is located. Doug Ischar calls to invite me to read in Chicago and when I tell him why it can't be until winter says YOU? in astonishment, perhaps the last lingering residual scrap of surprise at seeing an ex-teacher bounce down off whatever rickety pedestal he still keeps me on, and then FUCK FUCK FUCK many times, at various amplifications.

Fuck.

The question, says Kim over the last of yesterday's chicken soup, is not about bald but about all that hair you used to have.

TUESDAY | JULY 11, 2000

IN A MESSAGE DATED
7/11/00 JANECO WRITES:

i can say goodbye to your hair temporarily but i dont want to say goodbye to you.

IN A MESSAGE DATED
7/11/00 LDJOSE WRITES:

Don't forget the new relationship is not only with your hats, but more importantly with your pate. HAVE A DATE WITH YOUR PATE!!

Ed's office yesterday. The lump that appeared exactly where the tumor was is healthy new tissue. Don't worry. It's normal.

I feel like a freak, I say to my shrink. I have no style. I have no dignity. I'm marked. I'm a target. You don't look anything like that, she says, carefully. You look remarkable, it's true, but you look like a woman who has taken control.

It's fake, I say. It's a performance. Don't you get it? Can't you see? Are you blind?

Lunch with Susan S. There were people who wanted to hear about her big breakup, not her cancer. You figure out really fast who can behave like a friend and who can't. Susan doesn't make lists. I do.

WEDNESDAY | JULY 12, 2000

IN A MESSAGE DATED
7/12/00 LORRGRAD WRITES:

Yes, I have toes and fingers crossed for tomorrow. And look on the bright side. This time you won't wake up with hair in your mouth.

Meditate. When I come out the skin below my eyes is wet, but I can't say that I was crying.

IN A MESSAGE DATED
7/12/00 CBLORD@UCI.EDU
WRITES TO UNDISCLOSED
RECIPIENTS:

SUBJECT: THE LESBIAN PHALLUS

So far, in the way of coverings, now that I have lost my hair and ac-quired a pate, I have of course the Fred Segal black knit, or perhaps it is actually the darkest of navies, as well as a floppy brimmed canvas white, a gray blue watch cap, a dusky sage green knitted affair that looks to my mind a little too self deprecating, almost Smith and Hawkens in that white-woman-with-time-to-plant-peonies-behold-also-the-trowel-in-complementary-orange-see-page-fourteen look, a solid black base-ball cap, a red and black ZERO PATIENCE cap, water stained on the brim, a long ago gift from John Greyson, TWO Kangol black caps, like knitted baseball caps but minus the brim, very Che, except for the white kangaroo in front but then even though the whole world has gone brand nonetheless I do not think I can pull off Che even if I add a red ban-dana, a Target entirely synthetic hot pink fishing cap with black cow spots, a gift from Kim's ex, four black bandanas, one turquoise ban-dana, one military camouflage bandana, and the promise of a loan of a baseball cap, color unknown, that says JUST DO IT!

I have also acquired certain accessories (lipstick of a dark brownish red described as REVE DE MIEL, a XENA THE WARRIOR t shirt, and a silver and turquoise ear cuff). I have reevaluated my collection of neck-laces, most of them unworn, many of them gestures intended by my mother to fertilize the stunted signifiers of my femininity. Like color, which does not exist in isolation but is entirely determined by the adja-cent colors, the neck, which lies between breasts and head, is entirely changed by the deletion of hair and the addition of pate. Minus acces-sories, pate pretty much fills the entire visual field. No accessories means minimal going on victim. On a woman of my age pate spells invalid. InVAlid.

A shirt with a high collar helps. Also a V-neck. And a straight spine.

A few weeks ago, at the first meeting of my support group, I was asked to name my greatest fear. Going bald, I answered, without hesitation. Catherine, except for Louanne, who hasn't had chemo yet, most of us ARE bald, they explain. It hadn't dawned on me that they had gone to a store and bought what was covering their heads. I had thought they were amazingly well groomed for women who presumably felt like shit and in fact I felt a bit of unproductive and noxious superiority of the politically correct sort about the priority these middle-class women placed on appearances when faced with a life-threatening disease. Underneath this hat, said Suzie, lung cancer, the best-dressed woman in the group, it's baby orangutan, hairless with long wispy patches. If you want to FREAK people out, said Glenda, mother of two, the oldest ten, misread needle biopsy three years ago, double mastectomy and reconstruction—and now let us face it because she has, she is fucked, when my time is up my time is up, that's her mantra, and she has already talked to her children—if you want to FREAK people out, if you're at a party or a dinner or something and you want to REALLY freak them out, this is what you do. You say, it's so hot, I'm so hot I can't take it, and whip your wig off and throw it on a chair. Then you'll know who can deal.

Adriamycin was nothing, Glenda says. Taxol is awful.

So back to pate, which is, incidentally, prone to five o'clock shadow along the back and sides. Is there something worse than cancer for a middle-aged dyke? Could I have male-pattern baldness? Is pateness—stubble-free and silky—something I will have to WORK to maintain for the next five or six months? I have not grown accustomed to my pate, but in an odd and tentative dance, we are becoming acquainted. In order to walk down the street or into a restaurant or into a store, I must both remember my pate and forget that I have it. The memory in my muscles and the timbre of my voice carry me through interactions that used to be simple: asking for rice cakes in the health food store, returning a videotape, dropping off clothes at the cleaners. When you face your worst fear you crack and when you wake up you find out you're not dead, you're bald. The performance you do that is both you and the effect of you, the performance that teaches you who you are and who you can be and who you hope to be, that performance is only partly constructed by your hair, though of course you tend to believe that hair is its motive and necessary force. But my voice still works, along with my eyes, my humor, my stride. The performance performs the performer. If you don't let bald in, neither can other people. The performance will be thick enough to see me through. Collect the stares and use them later.

On the queer side of town, in Silver Lake, I've been reminded in an observation intended to be reassuring of the similarities between hats and dildos. As Cathy Opie once said of the latter, I love to use them but I'm glad they're removable. Personally, I know that Opie is not in actual fact the first person to float this boat, but now that the ship has sailed and she has left Los Angeles and gone to Yale to be a lesbian, as it were, it's understandable that she would get the credit for some celebrated recent theorizing about gender performance.

Q: Is hair as unnecessary a protrusion as a dick in most social circumstances? Conversely, is hair as much fun as a dick in most social circumstances?

Q: If the penis is located between the legs, and the phallus is located between the ears, where is a lesbian's hair when it is not on her head? (I have kept mine in zip-locked baggies, I confess, in anticipation of a future I do not yet understand, but this is a more literal answer than the sort I have in mind.)

Q: If a straight woman rushes to the wig store (get ready, get it in advance of the chemo, have it waiting so that it will be there when you need it . . .) what should a lesbian do? Wigs are tight. Wigs itch. Wigs are about passing. Or are wigs like lipstick? Get over it, apply the signifiers, hit the road.

Q: How come men OWN not only dicks but bald? In this year of the fabulous homeboy/dude/fag—take your pick of race and sexuality and combine as you will—how does a dyke lay claim to bald outside her own house?

Only my lover has so far seen my pate.

THURSDAY | JULY 13, 2000

Chemo Two. David will drive me to Cedars, Kim will meet me there and drive me home. I dread getting sicker but sick is an abstraction. I'm a cipher in other people's calculations of degeneration. The yardstick is fatigue. The translations are tired. It's no picnic. It will be a rough patch. It's the pits. The days will end earlier.

I am already exhausted.

My mother calls, to hover and to retreat at the same time, also to offer the only strategy she knows, which is to repeat that I will get through it.

SATURDAY | JULY 15, 2000

IN A MESSAGE DATED 7/15/00 KENM WRITES: It's a small world. I've heard. My mother had chemo and then they implanted something radioactive in her.

IN A MESSAGE DATED 7/15/00 WHYRAIN WRITES: JESUS Catherine, I always knew you were capable of the most Wittgensteinian ruminations, but baldness has apparently sent you into the philosophical ether. Losing a breast (even losing one's life?) hath no terrors equal to losing this first and last visible signifier of female virility. I remember years ago when I told Nancy Graves my hair was falling out and my mother had hardly any hair left at the end of her life, she said something to the effect that this was one thing that was just not "acceptable" for women. A huge no-no. And now that I've found a hair style that suits the inexorable genetic progress of hair erasure, it gives me pause to reflect on the whole megillah of pateness, as you put it. I see no reason for you to fret about showing your head. I fantasize feeling and kissing and patting it.

SUNDAY | JULY 16, 2000

IN A MESSAGE DATED 7/16/00 CBLORD@UCI.EDU WRITES TO UNDISCLOSED RECIPIENTS: SUBJECT: THE MAN WHO WAS ABSENT FROM THE FORUM OF HIS OWN DEVICES

Kim is meeting me at an expensive restaurant. The owner brings her to the back, which turns out to be her bedroom. The owner takes out a sex toy, a long green wiggly thing with a right angle in the middle and an elbow from which something red protrudes, like the flower on the orchid Kim had been watering yesterday afternoon. It was the most beautiful sex toy Kim had ever seen. The owner asked Kim to make love to her, so Kim began touching her breasts, but then she realized she couldn't fuck the woman because it would hurt me. Coincidentally, she noticed that the woman had no legs. Kim felt that the woman would take rejection hard, and so, with more than a bit of regret, as she was feeling very butch, she told the woman that she was waiting for her girlfriend. The good ones are always taken, said the woman. Then I came into the restaurant wearing a long cape with a hood that looked like long hair but when I pulled it back I had a very short cut underneath. I was more radiant than Kim had ever seen me. She watched heads turning as I moved through the room. When she looked back the restaurant woman had her legs again but she didn't have pubic hair.

It's your dream, I say, but it sounds to me like the old me versus the new me.

Whatever choice I made, it was still you, says Kim.

MONDAY | JULY 17, 2000

Baking soda baths. Alice down a long tunnel. Perhaps I should skip radiation and go back for a mastectomy. Whatever, Kim says. I'm not into normativity.

TUESDAY | JULY 18, 2000

IN A MESSAGE DATED
7/18/00 CBLORD@UCI.EDU
WRITES TO UNDISCLOSED
RECIPIENTS:

SUBJECT: WIG OUT

Wig out? reads the entirety of John Mason Kirby's reply to one of my emails. WIG OUT, I shoot back. A reminder that there might be a simple "solution" to my rantings? A question about whether the rantings indicate that I am in fact wigging out and should be fussed over in ways other than my appearance?

But wig is out. I have crossed off my list the possibility of a substitute, a fling, a replacement, a temporary solution that would imply a temporary problem. Not even a red nylon Cher mane. No hirsute dildos for Miss Natural. Somewhere back there, right after the lesbian haircut, wig went out, wig landed in the garbage, wig no longer tweaked the tender buttons, wig stayed on the store shelves. Wig would look wig, and cost plenty. (It is true that for a while, before the short haircut, I entertained the fantasy of a dread wig. I see now that this was an un-necessarily elaborate way to refuse in advance to pass.)

Wig was replaced by curiosity about my bare skull. More important, without being aware of any point at which I could be said to have made a decision, I realize that I want to be marked by baldness as a woman with cancer undergoing chemo, as a woman confronting her mortal-ity. In fact, before I noticed that the decision had arrived in me I was already marked. Something has been knifed inside me, and I do not want to lose the external sign of that wound.

I am in the profound place, Kim says, and though whenever there is a house with lights on by the side of the road, she promises to be in it, in truth I am on my own journey alone at dusk with my little kerchief of precious things.

Baldness is a scar. I want my scar. I want to be able to put my hands on it and have the wind touch it, to rub comfrey salve into it and to feel the rises and hollows of my skull without hair scratching and skidding under my fingertips. I don't want to shop to cover my scar, which will at any rate fade and heal, just as the ones on my breast and under my right arm are doing. I do not want to pass. I do not want to go gently back into the world of people who are afraid of looking into the eyes of someone whose chances of dying in the near future are better than theirs by a long shot, or so they need to believe. Baldness becomes me, in a literal sort of way, a hell of a lot better than a pink ribbon, though it is true that I now wear more jewelry. Here's the outfit for Chemo Two: black baggy pants, gray cotton knit pullover, black skull cap, bead bracelets. I understand now the woman in the pink jump suit and the strappy white sandals I stared at when I went for my first consultation with the illustrious Dr. Van Scoy Mosher. She was on her feet, holding it together, rummaging in her purse for her ten-dollar copayment, and she looked a lot better than the other people in the waiting room but her face was bright red after chemo and she didn't look good. I wanted to believe that wouldn't be me. I resolved never to wear pink to chemo.

You can only do the drag you know. She lives in Beverly Hills, or so I imagine, and I live Silver Lake.

IN A MESSAGE DATED 7/19/00 CROLLO WRITES: I think of Star Trek, Ionesco, and trolls, wish-nicks as we called them.

IN A MESSAGE DATED 7/19/00 CBLORD@UCI.EDU WRITES TO DEBOBR: i have absolutely no idea how you and jean managed it and i understand as i did not really then how abandoned you felt by me so if i couldn't really apologize before i do now. the isolation is intense.

IN A MESSAGE DATED 7/19/00 CBLORD@UCI.EDU WRITES TO SHARHA: Oi. My first cheese and (organic) tomato sandwich after a week, being tamped down with ginger tea as I write. It's slowly back to the land of the living, that is to say friends and tv and people who eat normal things and have normal lives. Speaking of TV, when are you coming to LA to watch cable?

The cup is half full, I suppose. People DO call, but I think they have a hard time realizing what this is actually like. Yesterday the lowest point: crying uncontrollably, thoughts of suicide, schemes to abandon treatment. Kim, otherwise known as Coach, came home to find me staring. THAT WON'T DO. I call Michael the oncologist, who clearly wants respect: title and last name. Please. I ask for something for aches and nausea. He pushes Advil. Chemo is just something you have to live through, he says. Eventually I extract Ativan.

I am exhausted.

THURSDAY | JULY 20, 2000

Nath calls from Marseille. Her father died of stomach cancer last year. She is dismantling her mother's house. You are loved, remember that at your worst moments.

Were you crying when you left the last time? I have a hard time accepting affection, I say to the shrink, like one of those dogs that just shivers and shakes and then howls or even snarls when you move in to make friends.

It's all about Catherine now, how Catherine feels, physically and emotionally, says Kim. There is no room for me.

IN A MESSAGE DATED
7/21/00 DEBOBR WRITES:

The strange thing about sojourning in the c-world is to discover who is there for you and who can't/doesn't deal. It's a deep irrational test of some sort and I never condemned anyone for not showing up.

IN A MESSAGE DATED
7/21/00 DHIJR WRITES:

Big hug.

IN A MESSAGE DATED
7/21/00 GENAB WRITES:

When my housing things are resolved and census kaput (very soon) i can probably ride a train across the big land again and visit . . . ok?

IN A MESSAGE DATED
7/21/00 CBLORD@UCI.EDU
WRITES TO UNDISCLOSED
RECIPIENTS:

SUBJECT: HER BALDNESS BECOMES AN ART COLLECTOR

Last Monday I received a gift of three garden sculptures from one of my graduate students. She has in the past fabricated covers for everyday objects ranging from guns to stacks of dishes to penises. More ambitiously and more recently, she has used thin plastic to construct full-scale models of symbolic architectural spaces that she inflates in locations such as fields and parking lots. Displacement.

The sculptures in question, however, Jennifer's one and only foray into the world of cement, were possibly something of an inconvenience. Two months ago, it seemed like the right thing to do. I was chair of Jennifer's thesis committee. I couldn't guarantee her fame, but I could give three small cement replicas of the internal space of her studio, each weighing four or five hundred pounds, a home as permanent as anyone can promise. I have a yard, of sorts. Why not accommodate the ghost of a teaching relationship? So what if it came to roost outside my bedroom window?

On Monday, Jennifer arrived, with Mario and Mark and Deirdre and a truck with an electrified ramp and dollies and ropes and carts. Nobody said a word about hair or its absence. Wobbly as I felt, sitting on the front porch propped against the wall, I realized that I was a spectacle and I made them afraid. I noticed that only one of them had thought to wear boots. I went inside to lie on the sofa, wonder what the liability limit is on my homeowner's insurance and skim one of the many lavender books I now own with the word BREAST in the title. Much crashing and sweating later, the sculptures were installed. Everyone went down to the back yard to pick plums except for responsible Deirdre, who stayed behind to fluff some of the plants that had been flattened by their encounter with concrete. I sat on the porch and watched her work. She wore a purple T shirt that said THE ONLY WAY TO WIN THE REVOLUTION IS GARDENING. For her final project, Deirdre turned a piece of nowhere above a drainage ditch in a Santa Ana barrio into a garden for neighborhood kids. It took them a year to find a patch of earth the city had forgotten to pave and plant a packet of sunflower seeds. They threw a big party. That was a week or so before I'd learned I had breast cancer.

Is chemo horrible? she asked.

Why, I wonder, is it unnerving to weep in front of a student? Even a graduated one? Even a slightly older one? Even a kind-hearted and somewhat scared one? Even a dyke? What would be the matter with a fair exchange? Their work, my tears. Why is weeping in a classroom, though we have all felt like it, more of a threat to the mortar that holds together the bricks than stupidity or hatred or ignorance?

You feel like shit, I say, face wet. Of course Deirdre hugs me. This is not quite right—the shit part, that is, not the hug part. Kristeva aside, I don't actually feel like a turd. Turd is a leap I cannot make. Nor do I feel like I have the flu, though the comparison is often volunteered. Flu feels like something is borrowing your body for nourishment. You don't want to make the loan but you can. Chemo is different. Something has broken into your body and it has murder on its mind.

Chemo is medieval, enough poison to make you crazy miserable but not enough to put you out of your misery. It's like a relic from the days when some people got to cover themselves in finely crafted metal skins while other people were crushed and pierced and slowly pulped. Lights are too bright, noises are too loud, your skin is not only too tight but much too thin, every pressure point in your body hurts, and so does your entire skull. The soles of your feet burn, everything going into your mouth, even the water that you must drink because you are desperately thirsty and because if you don't the drugs will sit in your bladder and corrode it from the inside out, everything feels like a bad idea.

Piss like a racehorse, the nurses tell you, and when you do, it comes out red. Though food on the face of it does not appear to be your friend you need something in your stomach besides water because when your stomach is empty you feel it beginning to consume itself. Nothing is funny, you can't read, you can't watch TV, you can't sleep and you cannot get the poison out of you because you have swallowed a pill that overrides the better instinct to vomit which you must avoid because you might seriously damage the lining of your stomach and esophagus. There are women who have described finding sheets of tissue in their puke.

Chemo is like mainlining weed killer, which is what, to invoke the perversely feminized metaphor oncologists prefer, my particular "recipe" sounds like. Adriamycin and Cytoxan: they fit right in on the pesticide shelf. You're not sure, however, whether you want to be picked for Team Crab or Team Bermuda and you would have much preferred to spend the entire game on the sidelines.

Chemo dosage is calculated by skin area. I have 1.7 square meters of skin. Morgan Fisher once happened upon the same chart my oncologist keeps in his desk drawer. Morgan used it to calculate his own skin area. He painted a rectangle exactly his size on a sidewalk in downtown Los Angeles and called it a self-portrait. To the best of my knowledge, Morgan has never had chemo.

There is in addition the matter of chemo brain, a phenomenon announced a few days ago by Canadian researchers. Chemo brain causes moderate to severe cognitive impairment, including memory loss, difficulty in concentration, and reduced logical function. Cancer patients have complained about chemo brain for decades, but doctors have only recently bothered to consider what weed killer might do to human brain cells.

On your worst days, you think that turds have it better, which is only to say that depression is one of the biggest side effects of chemo, it being difficult, let us face it, to keep up the chin, or the pecker, or the spirits, whichever you prefer, when you feel like a weed and perhaps, after all, not so very far from a turd. You have episodes of wondering why your sweetheart is spending two hours at the supermarket and where all your friends have gone and why your mother won't behave like a mother for once in her life and just get on a plane and why your therapist has forgotten to call and why even your cat has decided you are so boring she would rather sleep by herself.

The need for contact is voracious. After a week, you answer yes to every question on those checklists of symptoms to see whether you are A Depressed Person and should get professional help. Finally the legs get back the energy to climb out of the hole but the white blood count continues to drop. It does so for another two weeks, after which, all going well, it crawls back to a more or less normal level. You do, in fact, feel better in the short run, much better, but you also know that the weed killer is feasting on you and that any one of a list of unpleasant side effects could be in your future: heart attacks, kidney failure, intestinal parasites, collapsed veins, loss of sexual interest, sores in the rectum, skin so thin it splits, weight loss, weight gain, extreme fatigue, ditto vaginal dryness, olfactory hallucinations, severe skin burns, permanent hair loss, and, of course, the stress induced by waiting for the advent of any of the above. You begin to wonder. Is this how the end begins? The body, betrayed, no longer has confidence that what it takes in might nourish. Food doesn't fire the muscles. It saps them. You want nothing to penetrate the envelope of your skin. No feasting. No fucking.

On the same day you feel really and wonderfully human again, back to your old self, and happy, for a change, to be that old self, you're ready for the next round. Chemo works by killing all the fast-growing cells in your body, of which cancer is only one kind, the kind that cannot repair itself, or so the theory goes. That is to say, while other fast-growing cells repair themselves after chemo, cancer cells cannot. But when you stop to think about it, the difference between killing your fast-growing cells and killing you is a matter of splitting hairs and you are not in possession of hairs to split. This is what people are describing when they say that chemo brings you to death's door.

You bond with women who are going through the same thing. I know, for example, that Suzie's disability started two days ago. I know that she decided to shave off the final wisps of her baby orangutan hair last week, and that she hates looking in the mirror in the morning because before she looks, when she wakes up next to the guy she just married after living with him for seventeen years, she isn't a person with three more rounds to go. I know that Naomi, who has progressed from pate to fuzz, speaks from experience when she tells me not to worry about my blood count because whatever happens there is a drug that will take it back up again. I know that Glenda is going through Chemo Six today, and that her sister has come out from Georgia because it was so bad the last time Glenda's heart almost stopped and her ten year old daughter had to race for the nurse to take the drip out. Even though I don't really know Glenda I sit here writing and hope that she got back home safely and that I will see her next week.

How do you get through the depression? I asked my group last night. You just do, they say. People call you up. People bring you things. People take you out. You let people help. You let them do it now because they'll get bored with you later. There's a name for it. It's called compassion fatigue.

You weed, said Suzie, even if it's only for ten minutes. You just go out into the garden and weed.

SATURDAY | JULY 22, 2000

IN A MESSAGE DATED
7/22/00 SEC WRITES:

My mother went through this process. My brother, too. They were unable to articulate how it felt, so I really appreciate finally kind of understanding, or at least reading an effective description of it.

Glad the wig is out. Yes, show the scar! I mean, cross-dressing in my youth had some of that in it—fuck your fears of me, it said. At least partially, I get it. Here's another house on the side of the road with the lights on. Anything we can do we will do.

IN A MESSAGE DATED
7/22/00 JOEYS WRITES:

when you get a chance when you breath in let it enter your body and as you exhale let all the icky stuff exit. fill your heart with love. let me know when you're up for more company I'm here and I'm not going anywhere.

Susan R. calls. Fat means something different to her now. She wants substance.

My mother sends a get well card. Remember the woman who walked back from the Boiling Lake with a broken leg, she wrote. It will take all the courage you have, but you're strong enough to make it. When I call to thank her, she pulls back. You have to grit your teeth and get through it. You're lucky. You've been very healthy. So have I.

Vein hurts. I can see the bruise under the skin. My throat scratches and my eyes are dry but I am hoping it will be better next time with the burdock and the slippery elm.

IN A MESSAGE DATED 7/22/00 CBLORD@UCI.EDU WRITES TO UNDISCLOSED RECIPIENTS:

SUBJECT: HER BALDNESS MEETS JULIA MARIE

There have been many gifts. A beautiful pesto dinner by the front door at an especially dismal moment, a loaf of bread, books and books and books, rides and offers of rides, movie dates, lunches, dinners, hats, bandanas, a paperweight with a moose inside, offers to read out loud. Here's another.

My friend Annie, who is working to grow a new love in San Francisco, left town for a week or so. On Wednesday night she sent me a woman called Julia Marie. She advised me that Julia Marie was subtle, and asked me to give her a chance. Julia Marie unfolded her table while I sat nervously in the armchair, naked under my T shirt and baggy cotton pants, but of course wearing my little black cap, dreading the prospect of peeling it off for a stranger.

What kind of massage do you do?

She finished unfolding and walked over to me. I believe that there's a blueprint for each of us that was drawn before we were born, even before we were conceived, and that afterwards, as we live and change, we deviate from our blueprint. My job is to show you the blueprint, which is what is right about you, so that you yourself can choose to return to it. I do this by manipulating the cranio sacral fluid. When I do my deepest work sometimes I don't even touch people.

I begin to worry in advance about this encounter. I decide to be Proactive About My Needs. My whole right shoulder hurts, I say, all along the part where a wing would attach, if I had one, and I badly need a massage. A classic massage. A deep massage.

I don't want to see my blueprint in a mirror. I want it not to hurt where it hurts so that I can sleep through the night. I don't say this part out loud.

OK, says Julia Marie, but I'll give you an idea of what you're missing. She's quite small, she's wearing pressed linen shorts, her sandals are not hip, she doesn't go to a gym. The little black cap pulls off with my T shirt, making Julia Marie the third person to see my pate, after Kim and after Michelle, the nurse in the oncologist's office who drips the weed killer into the vein of my left arm and who is getting a divorce from her doctor husband because she has learned in her line of work that life is too short not to do what you want to do. Julia Marie has small hands. They heat the oil she uses before it even hits my body. They are so hot they startle. They are hot whether they are on my skin or whether they are half an inch away, cupping the air to follow the shape of my shoulder blade or the side of my neck or the plane of my temple. She works EXTREMELY slowly, drawing long inexorable lines. Her hands push the lines into my muscles and the knots inside feel like speed bumps. She starts at the bottom of my spine and moves up along my back to the base of the shoulder blade and then over the rotator along my arm. She makes it all connect, so that I can feel my shoulder blade as the mid point between the base of my spine and my finger tips. First she does the right side, the cancer side, the cut side, then she does the left, then my neck and skull, the backs of my legs, then the fronts and finally my chest and belly.

This is not a sexual experience. Neither is it erotic. My body is being read. My ex cherie's grandmother used to find truffles in the south of France by watching how flies circled and buzzed until they finally returned to light on a particular spot of soil. Howard Snow, a fisherman I once had a thing about, could stand on the prow of his boat in the middle of Cape Cod bay and point beneath the waves to the line where his oyster beds ended and where his neighbor's began. I am being gauged. Imagine the fingertips of a climber patting the rock face above her head to fathom the indentation that will give purchase, or the way a vine knows through its tendrils the air in the crevices of a stone wall, or the way an archaeologist might taste her find.

The left side of my body hurts more acutely than the side I had expected to hurt, the right side, the cut side. There, on the cancer side, the pain feels at once smaller in its location and vast in its hollowness, as if it were so ancient that it had forgotten the reason it left home and began to hunt for sustenance elsewhere. Julia Marie sits in a chair at the head of the massage table and covers, somehow, the entire top of my head—and my head was, humiliatingly so in Burlington, Iowa in 1966, the largest head in the entire graduating high school class, larger than the largest football player's head—somehow Julia Marie covers the entire top of my head with her two small hands.

I don't usually get to say this to people, she says, or I think she says, as she is whispering, but you have a beautiful head. An uncertain interval later she removes her hands, one at a time, first the left and then the right. A tremendous coolness lifts from my scalp.

I think about asking her to move in with us. She has run a pool hall in Bakersfield, sold real estate, managed a gourmet catering business, and produced floral arrangements. Everything makes sense except the real estate. I'd like to make you a gift she said, I'll come back and show you what I really do.

OK.

SUNDAY | JULY 23, 2000

IN A MESSAGE DATED 7/23/00 EBIRR WRITES: Through several mutual friends I hear that you are going through an ordeal of the medical type. I am just writing to say that I am thinking about you and hope your spirits are good and your health rebounds quickly. I am sure you have great support, but even so, if you need an ear, either of mine is available.

IN A MESSAGE DATED 7/23/00 CBLORD@UCI.EDU WRITES TO SEC: Why is it that the houses with the lights on always belong to people who have been through it themselves in one way or another? While we're on the subject of frailty, didn't you just have a doctor's appointment?

IN A MESSAGE DATED
7/24/00 CATGUN WRITES:

i'm sending you all of my love vibes and i'm sorry you're having to go through this. really sorry. especially about the depression.

love you love you love you i do i do i do

Lunch with Daniel. People hear it's life-threatening and rumors fly, but you're just you.

I am more at ease bald in the world. The week seems busy. Strong enough to weed.

I worry that I am being transformed by the intensity of my life while Kim stays in the same place. As soon as my body feels better life slides back to normal. I feel both more and less fear of death. I try to imagine death but cannot yet arrive at the moment breathing stops. Like Zeno's runner, my mind never reaches the target. Half there, and then half there again.

IN A MESSAGE DATED
7/24/00 CBLORD@UCI.EDU
WRITES TO UNDISCLOSED
RECIPIENTS:

SUBJECT: RECENT ACCESSIONS, COLLECTION OF HER BALDENSS
Black Uncle Jer's hat identical to the black Fred Segal's but which cost half as much even NOT on sale

Black wool skull cap, well used, with Nike swoosh and JUST DO ME

Faded burgundy fishing cap with JUST DO IT

Crocheted white skull cap

White cotton summer fez with gold stitching

Embroidered maroon fez with mirror inlays

Blue baseball cap with FIER D'ETRE MARSEILLAIS

TUESDAY | JULY 25, 2000

IN A MESSAGE DATED
7/25/00 CATGUN WRITES:

Page 47, "People in Review," *Art in America Annual*, 2000–2001. If I knew this serious-looking woman to the left of Elizabeth Murray, I might have a conversation with her that goes something like this: Why do you want all that hair? What good is it doing you? Everyone has hair. Mather schmather.

SUBJECT: HER BALDNESS GETS SOMETHING OFF HER CHEST

Julia Marie asks me to lie on my back with my eyes closed. Her hands cup the air above my ankles. Then she moves to my skull, after which she moves to the base of my spine, placing one hand under my back and the other very lightly on that part of my torso directly above her hand. She moves the bottom hand up slightly. She places the other hand on my lower belly, then on the right pelvic bone, then on the left. It feels like a pond, I tell her. Your hands are resting on the banks. There's a tightness in the center, a turbulence rising in the middle. She moves the bottom hand to my thoracic vertebrae and puts the top hand lightly on the center of my chest at the place where the ribs join. She stays. Cold fear rises, the distinct feeling of feet sitting on my chest, yellow hairless animal feet, possibly bird, at any rate a bitter cold damp weight, something waiting and spreading and settling. Julia Marie stays there a long time. Her hands are hot but it is forever before they warm me. Finally she puts one hand under the base of my neck and the other on my throat. It's all pain in the shoulders and neck and jaw until finally heat runs down sheets of muscle, down my arms down the front of my body down my back.

Shaman, I keep saying to myself. Endure because it will make you stronger. Endure because it will temper you. Go through fire and come out the other side. If you melt metal in a crucible the molecular structure changes so that it can tolerate greater heat. It seems ridiculously macho. A sweat lodge. Clear air and red rock and thunderstorms. I want them.

There was a vacuum in your chest, Julia Marie says later, two hours later. It pulled my hand into your chest. Usually I don't apply that much pressure.

She hasn't massaged a single muscle of my body, but I come out with barely an ache, completely energized, wanting to giggle, ravenous, wanting to get on with it, not to waste time, to move forward fast and clean.

Near the end, Kim comes home. She feels like such an interloper she doesn't notice the flowers I have brought her. Maybe Julia Marie is the deep thing you're doing right now, she says. Maybe it's not verbal.

I wake at 4 A.M. The dream camera is zooming back from a stormy green sea, waves foaming, across which the tiny speck of a boat is moving. The boat is only paper, but it is moving steadily forward.

WEDNESDAY | JULY 26, 2000

Little flecks of stubble when I rub my pate. Mouth sores. Vein still bruised.

Shrink notes that a month ago I couldn't even get a haircut. Are you suicidal? I think about killing myself for the first three or four days after chemo, I reply, but I'm too sick to get it together. She wonders if they are giving me steroids. Depression can be a side effect. I call Michael, excuse me, Dr. Van Scoy Mosher. I am indeed getting steroids with the chemo. A few other women have said it made them depressed, he observes, but he doubts the depression is actually an effect of the drug.

Matias calls. Everything is about how to get rid of illness, or how to cure it, he says. Nothing is about how just to have it.

IN A MESSAGE DATED 7/26/00 CBLORD@UCI.EDU WRITES TO UNDISCLOSED RECIPIENTS:

SUBJECT: EPISODES IN THE UNVEILING OF HER BALDNESS
You know about Kim, because, after all, she is my lover and she pated me. I have also told you about Michelle, the oncologist's nurse in the process of getting a divorce who mentioned in passing that she doesn't see the pates of most women she treats because they never remove their hats or wigs in the office. Some women, she is certain, never remove their wigs at home. She thinks most women would rather lose a breast, or both breasts, than lose their hair. I've told you about Julia Marie, reformed real estate agent. These private viewings were followed by a collective unveiling in my support group last week when three of the four bald women decided to show their stuff, led by Glenda, of course, who JUST DID IT, followed by Suzie and then Her Baldness, who had to put her money where her mouth was since she had started the whole conversation by asking questions about who in our lives had actually seen our pates. So there we were, applauding ourselves but maybe after the noise had died down feeling a little bare in front of each other, not to mention the therapist and the woman training to set up a cancer center in Japan, and the other therapist in training to work somewhere else, who is learning so much from us, like not to change the subject when people want to talk about cancer, and Louanne, who is neither an observer nor a facilitator but a woman with cancer who

has managed, what with one thing and another, to miss the first six or so of her scheduled chemo treatments. Sometimes she can't get a ride. Sometimes she wants to change doctors. Sometimes it's just not a good moment. Sometimes her insurance company messes up. Sometimes she needs to do more research. Louanne used to teach kindergarten. Last week she threw out all the materials she'd accumulated in twenty years of teaching. Louanne is terrified.

We agreed that pate viewing is a privilege, not a right. Tests of constancy and sincerity and general helpfulness are in order. You don't put out for anyone on the first visit, that's for sure, certainly not for the one-off sort of visitor who wants to eyeball someone on their way out. When they say, I'm so sorry you have this, says Glenda, they really mean, I'm SO glad I don't.

Why do men get to own bald? I asked the group, hoping for simple answers to big questions. Because they just naturally go bald, suggested the substitute facilitator, a man. If you think about the statistics, I retort, one in seven, or one in eight, and then figure that if even a third of these women get chemo, then there are a lot of bald women out there who are completely invisible as a class. And that's for breast cancer alone. One in three Americans get some kind of cancer.

But as it turns out, despite our bravery in stripping for each other, not one of us has gone bald outside the safety of our houses. Well, once I forgot and went out in the morning to grab the newspapers, but then I dashed back in, looking over my shoulder and feeling like an idiot. So much for organizing the Bald Brigade. Anyway, my question divided the room into teams: besides the two abstainers—Geraldine, who chose not to remove her wig, and Louanne, who hasn't yet lost her hair—it was three bald women versus three hairy social workers. For a minute there, hair looked big and dry and pointless, as nasty and stupid as tumbleweed. If hair is really the phallus which has been disguised as a fetish for a few centuries, Team Helping Professions dropped the dildo and Team Cancer slid it in gently from downtown.

The next morning, when Kim and I went to see the shrink, I whipped off the black cap and the shrink, bless her, said WOW, and borrowed my camera to take pictures, which I think in some way enabled me to strip for Annie when she came for a visit in the afternoon, a nervous moment between friends, I must say. It would be easier to have sex with Annie because then at least there would have been a script of sorts. Annie too said WOW, so I modeled Her Baldness's Collection, Department of Hats, and we settled on the crocheted white Algerian skull cap for a brunch the next day, a smallish affair with people who knew but with whom I hadn't spoken, a cap which says YOU CAN SEE PERFECTLY WELL THROUGH THE HOLES THAT I AM BALD AND IN THIS CASE IF ORNAMENT IS CRIME YOU'RE THE PERPETRATOR.

After that it's been mainly back to the skull caps, all rolled up so that they sit on the top of my head and you can see the back of my skull, from which, by the way, it being day fourteen, I notice that stubble is just beginning to fall again. I am finding tiny little black flecks on my palms. Her Baldness is getting over herself, she is, liking to rub her hands over the scratchy parts of her scalp, liking the afternoon breeze on the back of her neck, feeling fashionably modernist as an object, getting acquainted with the ears she kept hidden for the entire last half of the twentieth century, imagine that, and realizing that though her entire self-appointed existence as an honorific is a blatant displacement of her fear of mortality on the other hand the third person is a good one when code is the only way to speak about what nobody wants to say.

THURSDAY | JULY 27, 2000

Blood count 2,900, burning pee. Nutritionist gives me stuff for the kidneys and says, after taking her usual digs at the medical profession, that I look in astoundingly good shape. Make an appointment with radiation oncologist. Looking to put a marker between sickness and health, I find a silent retreat in Massachusetts. When I tell Kim, she is disappointed. She wants to be together after all my treatments. OK. I don't need to run to the other side of the country to be still.

IN A MESSAGE DATED 7/27/00 CBLORD@UCI.EDU WRITES TO UNDISCLOSED RECIPIENTS:

SUBJECT: RECENT ACCESSIONS, COLLECTION OF HER BALDNESS, DEPARTMENT OF GETTING ON WITH IT

It will grow back.

It will grow back without the gray.

Show the scar.

It will grow back curly.

It's a gift to have someone unadorned, naked, living her or his life bald, right there in front of you.

You can pull off Che.

It will grow back straight.

Maybe there's a kind of utopian pleasure to shedding the phallus (or is that something only a relatively affluent white male can say?).

By the time it grows back you won't want it.

It might grow back a different color.

You have great bones.

You can get away with it.

People might think you're a Buddhist nun.

Look at all those toupees.

You've turned into a hip chick.

Sigourney Weaver was fucking hot without hair.

Experience is the comb that nature gives us when we are bald.

FRIDAY | JULY 28, 2000

IN A MESSAGE DATED 7/28/00 JMK WRITES:

Owning bald is about as rewarding as owning a piece of land that's ten feet under (piranha infested) water. One boy's view: you bald girls are ok.

If I didn't have such a fat head and fatter round fat face then I would do it because my hair is completely gray and it doesn't go with my Clearasil complexion so I keep dying it every two weeks and it falls out in huge dry piles everywhere and I spend several minutes a day scooping it up and thinking, yup, I'm making myself lose my hair and my brain cells because I'm vain.

Linda's fiftieth birthday today. She is celebrating quietly with her friend Louise, shopping for the little things she likes to buy, my sad little sister with a big heart who has just sent me a subscription to Yoga Journal.

Lunch with Annie. We talk about sex and shame. Alicia B. wanders up. She doesn't ask. I don't tell.

SATURDAY | JULY 29, 2000

Remember, I'm only a flight away—and Jennifer said she would give me a good reference. She also said—Catherine? No problem. She's as stubborn as I am.

SUNDAY | JULY 30, 2000

One of our old Saturdays: yoga, errands, Eames show, Barney's, beach walk, or rather beach sit, dinner, and a video at home. Her Baldness is less sorry for herself today. Truth is that when I feel better—physically strong and OK about my appearance—I don't want to think about death or chemo. Truth is also that when I feel better I forget the side effects of weed killer. All I have to remind me today is a bald head and knots under the skin in the crook of my arm.

Her Baldness is getting full of herself.

MONDAY | JULY 31, 2000

I've been thinking for months that I'd like to see a sparks game. I was hoping that if I could get tickets, you might want to come.

IN A MESSAGE DATED
7/31/00 DEBOBR WRITES: So "most women" would rather lose breasts than hair, eh? I wonder if they feel that way after the hair grows back, which it does. We're alive, dammit. That's beauty enough.

Chemo Three on Thursday. Three and a half weeks until the last one. Four and a half weeks until the worst of the effects, knock mouse on the wooden desk top, are over. I make the list. What if a blood clot floats off? What if I have to have one of those ports surgically implanted in my chest? What if Kim leaves me? What if Linda doesn't do the dishes?

Immense slothfulness, like frostbite. It scratches when I turn my head on the pillow. Soft down is growing back amongst the stubble.

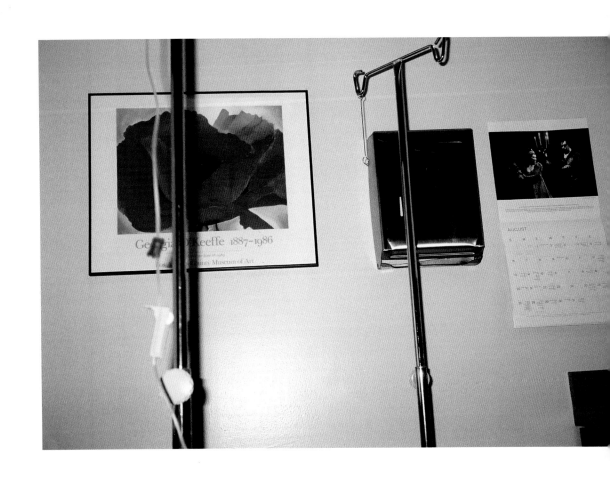

AUGUST | 2000

IN A MESSAGE DATED
8/1/00 GENAB WRITES:

To Her Baldness, c/o complaint department: do you send ONLY "mass emails" now?

Chemo prep. Grapefruit juice, watermelon juice, bread, sardines. Cat food and the Tibetan Book of Living and Dying, *Pema Chodron on Tonglen meditation. Annie comes to tell me she's going to San Francisco tomorrow for the rest of the month. I am bereft.*

IN MESSAGE DATED
8/1/00 CBLORD@UCI.EDU
WRITES TO UNDISCLOSED
RECIPIENTS:

SUBJECT: HER BALDNESS GOES BACK TO SCHOOL

Normally, as a fifty-one-year-old woman, my risk of developing breast cancer would be somewhere between 1 in 50 at age fifty and 1 in 33 at age fifty-five. (By age eighty, should we be so lucky, the risk is 1 in 10.) Susun Weed's Breast Cancer Risk Assessment Test, found at the back of her book *Breast Cancer? Breast Health! The Wise Woman Way,* is designed to measure factors causing risk increase against factors causing risk reduction. Risk here means the chance of developing breast cancer, not of dying from breast cancer, though naturally the former increases the risk of the latter.

RISK INCREASES IN MY CASE

My waist to hip ratio is above .81	+60
I never gave birth	+55
I smoked commercial cigarettes regularly	+40
I had regular mammograms before menopause	+40
My ancestors are Caucasian and I have light skin	+30
I am taller than 5' 3" and weigh more than 154 pounds	+30
I am a lesbian	+30
Both grandmothers had breast cancer	+25
I use a TV or computer monitor more than 20 hours weekly	+20

I shower in chlorinated water	+10
I soak in chlorinated water an hour a week	+10
I often stay up late with electric lights on	+10
I frequently feel resentful	+10
I chew on my feelings	+10
I don't feel appreciated	+10
I began menstruating at age 12	+ 8
I am a teacher, librarian, or religious worker	+ 3
I use a chemical deodorant	+ 3
I lived in North America between 1961 and 1963	+ 2
(it would have been +14 had I lived in North America between 1949 and 1961)	
I used estrogen replacement for six months	+.5
I do not regularly shave the hair from my armpits	+ 0
TOTAL RISK INCREASE	+406.5

RISK DECREASES IN MY CASE

My grandparents ate mostly organic food	-50
I set aside regular time to relax	-20
I eat three cups of fruit/vegetables a day	-15
I have exercised 20 minutes 3 times a week for 15 years	-15
I eat three or more servings of whole grains daily	-10
I have ways to be with my pain and my anger	-10
I eat iodine-rich foods regularly	- 5
I've had a suspicious lump in my breast biopsied	- 0
I eat an even-caloried diet that is 30% or less fat	- 0
TOTAL RISK DECREASE	-125

Doing further calculations particular to Susun Weed's system, the details of which I'll spare you, means that my chances of developing breast cancer at my age doubled from almost 2% to almost 4%. That's the risk factor of a woman of sixty.

Almost half of my risk increase, or 205 points, comes from being a tall, childless, light-skinned lesbian getting thick around the middle in her fifty-first year. Make that a lesbian who took care of herself by getting mammograms more or less regularly and it brings it up to 245 points.

Look at it another way: being a white, conscientious, childless dyke has cost me ten years.

Getting those mammograms, combined with reading at night, neutralizes my grandparents' eating habits. Alternately, not that it's of any current functional value, my grandparents' eating habits more than offset either my being a neurotic, tormented, under-appreciated gnawer of feelings or my smoking like a chimney for twenty years.

Eating fish does not offset using deodorant and being a teacher, but it does take care of immigrating to the U.S. in 1961.

Eating fruit and vegetables does not offset using a computer.

Long baths with the lights on neutralize the effect of minimizing stress by relaxing in long baths with the lights on.

Having a suspicious lump in my breast biopsied (and found to be benign, in the other breast, two years ago) makes as little difference as not bothering to shave my armpits.

WEDNESDAY | AUGUST 2, 2000

IN A MESSAGE DATED
8/2/00 HEYLORD WRITES:

Maybe I should put a chlorine filter on our showerhead.

IN A MESSAGE DATED
8/2/00 CROLLO WRITES:

OK, what about reading books? Is that a negative or a positive factor? Advanced degrees? (I think I already know that.) Oh, and how can I forget, what about faculty meetings? Those must put at least as much risk on you as smoking or refusing to birth babies. I wish there were formulas for more upbeat things than breast cancer. I'd like to know what my chances are for writing a successful book.

When I tell Kim I want to take care of financial arrangements, she weeps and I get furious. I want her to face things, not live in illusion and denial. We'll never have a child OR a puppy, she says. You couldn't take the stress.

IN A MESSAGE DATED
8/2/00 CBLORD@UCI.EDU
WRITES TO UNDISCLOSED
RECIPIENTS:

SUBJECT: INVENTORY, COLLECTION OF HER BALDNESS,
DEPARTMENT OF HOPE

Cedar smoke
Banana smoothies
Milk shakes
Watermelon juice
Water
Ice cubes (dry throat)
Moisturizing cream
Warm compress (bruised vein)
Cold compress (bruised vein)
St. John's wort oil (radiation burn)
Seaweed (radiation)
Brown rice
Rice
Green leafy vegetables
Ativan (anxiety)
Zofran (nausea)
Kytril (nausea)
Valium (anxiety)
Marinol (can't remember)
Advil (muscle pain)
Wormwood
Slippery elm
Burdock root
Calcium
Vitamins (A, E, C, B complex)
Selenium
Arnica
Salmon
Tofu
Acupuncture
Meditation
Visualization
A puppy
A kitten
A child
Chicken soup
Ginger tea
Liquid tears

IN A MESSAGE DATED
8/3/00 GENERAB WRITES:
give a signal/sign when you are UP and ABOUT with appetite again for all . . . ok?

IN A MESSAGE DATED
8/3/00 CBLORD@UCI.EDU
WRITES TO UNDISCLOSED
RECIPIENTS:
SUBJECT: HER BALDNESS COUNTS CHICK PEAS AND
NEW POTATOES

If you get the highest possible score on Susun Weed's pluses for increased risk exam it doesn't mean you WILL develop breast cancer. Conversely, if you get the highest possible score on the decreased risk column—those of you who have been pregnant a lot, never taken birth control or eaten meat, slept outdoors away from electricity at least two nights per year, do regular breast exams, don't hold grudges, love yourselves no matter what, and are willing to ask for what you want—it doesn't mean that you WON'T develop breast cancer.

This is what turned up at the end of May. A gritty, irregular, white, diffuse mass, infiltrating ductal carcinoma, poorly differentiated (histologic grade 3, nuclear grade 3, estrogen receptor negative, her2neu expressed) 1.7 cm x 1.5 cm x 1.5 cm in the 12 o'clock position of my R Breast, and in addition one of 29 dissected lymph nodes positive for metastatic carcinoma. The involvement of the lymph nodes and the size of the tumor make my diagnosis early Stage II cancer, on a ladder with four rungs.

Had I declined chemo, my approximate survival rate, according to Dr. Susan Love, would be 70-85% for five years and 45-55% for ten years. Chemo increases my chances to 85-90%. I am taking a stronger course of chemo (specifically, Adriamycin and Cytoxan) because, according to my oncologist, that increases my odds by two or three percent over CMF, the milder course, relatively speaking, where conceivably I might not have lost my hair. I could be one of ninety survivors, with hair, or one of 93 survivors, without hair. The three extra bald women make all the difference. I imagine us getting together somewhere to drink gallons of anti-oxidant green tea (perhaps we'd camp out for a few nights, away from electricity) and discuss the invasion of the medical profession by food metaphors.

Her Baldness has been getting out and about lately, in between her second and third infusion of weed killer, on what I would call the normal course of errands in a Los Angeles summer, that is, meals in the hood, movies, errands to the grocery store, hardware store, bookstore, vet, pharmacy, photo lab, video store, the usual. She has managed to avoid all art openings and parties, but she has gotten herself to a museum or two on quiet days. Her Baldness generally comes into existence on the other side of the front door, though the question of whether to let Her Baldness out arises when friends come into the privacy of my house. So far, apart from Julia Marie and Michelle and the women in my support group, I am completely comfortable only with Kim and Annie. I can imagine working up to it with a few other people, at home, but haven't yet. My little sister Linda is coming on Monday, however, and that will be another person. I can't imagine wearing a hat around her, nor can I imagine that she would wish me to do so.

Her Baldness, aspiring to Her Boldness, feels content with a quiet life in the neighborhood and an occasional trip to the beach. She does her yoga, working up to about ten sun salutations and all the standing poses except twisting triangle which she avoids, as she always has, except under group pressure. She reads, most lately about monasteries. She's always wanted to go to one, to Kim's chagrin, or said she did. She has in mind reading novels with occasional breaks for Gregorian chants sung by people who can carry a tune and eating good vegetarian meals without having to wash a single dish. Her Baldness is living in her own private monastery at the moment (watch what you wish for) but she has in mind something more structured, feeling that at the moment it's all about confronting matters of life and death and meaning, and she wants to be with other people who have the same interests, even though this sounds like a cliché and no one wants to be exactly where she is. She's realized that she can't actually do the Christian version, for reasons philosophical as well as pragmatic, so she is flirting with Buddhism, about which she knows little, having always been suspiciously anti-religious. (Remember, we're not talking about Her Boldness.) Nonetheless, right now two things appeal: the idea of concrete strategies that would still the mind when it hurts AND the idea of a philosophy that, seeing life as the mirror of death, requires that you become familiar with death. (But, says Pema Chodron, when you first start meditation you think that when you've calmed the turbulence all will be beauty and instead, you see through clear water to all the trash at the bottom of the pond.) Her Baldness hasn't managed to sit still for longer than half an hour. Breathe in the pain, breathe out compassion. Whatever you are feeling, other people feel the same.

Though she may turn up elsewhere and otherwise, Her Baldness was born of shame. Eve Sedgwick mentions, in her book *Dialogue on Love*, her simple shame, during her chemo for breast cancer, at being a freak— a 250 pound, soft spoken, SMART bald woman. There's the grotesquerie of being excessively vulnerable in public space, even if that public space is inside your own private house, in fact even if the very naming of your house as "private" means that logically it is precisely the opposite. There's the shame of being marked. There's the shame of having flunked some test and gotten sick (incapable of dealing with stress, too much repressed anger, all those cigarettes, all that alcohol, the bad breakup, bad genes, etc.). There's shame about being the junker stalled on the shoulder while all the fancy new models speed by.

I'm used to being a winner in the statistics game, the top 10% or 5% or 1% or 0.1% of whatever the field is but suddenly I'm in the bottom 10% or so for having gotten breast cancer in the first place and potentially in the bottom 8 or 10% of that bottom 10% if the treatments don't work and the new potatoes multiply. On the other hand, I could already have been cured by surgery, and the chemo and radiation might be unnecessary. It's a crap shoot, and my hunch is that even crap shoots have more predictability than this particular dance of subatomic particles. There's the shame at the surface of my confused pate. My hair follicles seem not to know whether they are in the middle of living or dying. My pate is a mixture of black stubble frozen in time, smooth skin, and, though very sparse, the finest and blondest of downy hair growing wild like lupine after a forest fire.

Susan Love says that the only way you know you're cured of cancer is if you live long enough to die of something else.

The costume for my third chemo: beige linen pants, gray camisole, black bra, wrinkled white shirt, crocheted cap, silver bracelet.

IN A MESSAGE DATED
8/4/00 KTHOM WRITES:
I love Her Baldness/Boldness. I want her to go to a monastery, if she wants to. I want her to sleep outside away from electricity with me. I want her to never feel shame, especially over a little cell mutation, but I do understand. Mostly I want her to live such a long and healthy life that she actually forgets the year she had cancer. She is most definitely more bold than bald.

TUESDAY | AUGUST 8, 2000

IN A MESSAGE DATED
8/8/00 JMK WRITES:
I like those three extra bald women, too. You never know when having an extra bald woman around will come in handy.

WEDNESDAY | AUGUST 9, 2000

IN A MESSAGE DATED
8/9/00 GENAB WRITES:
PLEASE, please give a signal/sign that you are okay . . . would REALLY appreciate THAT very much.

Queasies worse, fatigue better, and sweet to have Linda here, puttering, gentle, undemanding. Another fear gone.

Phone has been ringing: Susan S., Sharon, Jane, warm and funny though I cannot remember the substance, Annie, Betty, Ann S., Susan Cahan with news of $7,500 from the Norton Foundation to work on the Dominica book. Thank you, I say, that is wonderful news. I can't get to it right now, but I will go to work as soon as I can. I doze and when I wake I want it all to be worth it.

FRIDAY | AUGUST 11, 2000

IN A MESSAGE DATED
8/11/00 DEBOBR WRITES:
Cytoxan/cyclophosphamide, as I'm sure you know by now, was the active agent in mustard gas of Great War fame. When you close your eyes, do you hear the shells screaming in and feel the mud splattering as they carpet-bomb your cells?

SUNDAY | AUGUST 13, 2000

IN A MESSAGE DATED
8/13/00 CBLORD@UCI.EDU
WRITES TO JEANNIEW:
I'd love to see you too, as I need a friends break, but I have a bit of bad news, which is that I was diagnosed with breast cancer at the end of May and have been doing chemo this summer and will be doing radiation in the fall. It's early, prognosis good, etc., etc., but it's a hard thing.

IN A MESSAGE DATED 8/13/00 CBLORD@UCI.EDU WRITES TO MMORGAN:	Thanks for the thoughts. The thing about this is that there are no plans.
IN A MESSAGE DATED 8/13/00 CBLORD@UCI.EDU WRITES TO CWOLF:	It's my first morning back at the computer. One more round.
IN A MESSAGE DATED 8/13/00 CBLORD@UCI.EDU WRITES TO JOANA:	I'm so sorry. Nancy Naples told me that you had been diagnosed with ovarian cancer.

Kim rents Errol Morris's Dr. Death. I cannot bear to watch a man explain how to kill other men more efficiently. You were the one who said she wanted to see it, Kim says. She and Linda give me first choice of all the leftovers. Am I too thin? I ask, realizing suddenly how baggy my pants have become. No, they say, not really. No, not at all. Don't worry.

MONDAY | AUGUST 14, 2000

IN A MESSAGE DATED 8/14/00 LDJOSE WRITES:	A quick message to say 1) I'm thinking of you and 2) I did bring you a rock from Macchu Picchu.

Linda gone. Heavy. Nausea. Weakness therefore depression. I feel the blood count crashing. Three months of unbalanced checkbooks. When things fall apart they fall fast. I root around for the strength that was there just this morning. I am afraid of the tiredness itself. Cancel shrink appointment. Just one more chemo, she says. I like her less and less.

Kim's mother calls to chat. Everyone she knows has cancer. Everyone she knows has had chemo. Everyone she knows goes to chemo alone. Some people drive themselves to chemo, sixty miles and back. Kim's mother is jealous.

I do not have the strength to repel the stares. Why am I embarrassed? Who gives a fuck? Why is it so hard to see the scalp of a middle-aged woman?

TUESDAY | AUGUST 15, 2000

Not even Ativan. Dominica so far away.

IN A MESSAGE DATED
8/16/00 ANNEJUN WRITES:

feeling any better? less tired? when are you going to take a little get-away together?

IN A MESSAGE DATED
8/16/00 CBLORD@UCI.EDU
WRITES TO UNDISCLOSED
RECIPIENTS:

SUBJECT: WHAT'S HER BALDNESS BEEN DOING ALL THIS TIME?
A few nights ago I got stoned, as munchies do indeed help nausea, and Kim and I took my little sister Linda, who had come from Florida for a week to help us, to a fancy restaurant in Pasadena to celebrate Linda's fiftieth, which has been put off due to the BrCa diagnosis. Lo and behold, seated at the very next table was another pate—hatless, younger, smaller, prone to turquoise in the tank tops, and far enough along to be quite thin in the eyebrow department—out for a special dinner with her adoring boyfriend. In the middle of all the rich white Pasadena family folk, HB suddenly felt overdressed and also rather like a teletubby. She wanted to wobble and jig and wave and open her eyes wide and burble. PAT PAT YUM. No luck. No meaningful eye contact. No cancer bonding. No recognition. Not even a little twitch at the corner of the lips. So HB folded up her purple triangle and ordered raw tuna and arugula and fish piled on polenta and a dessert involving astonishing amount of butterfat and sugar, all of which she downed with gusto, her first real meal in ten days.

Before that, it was a lot of sleeping, aided by Ativan, Tammy Faye Baker's drug of choice. (Perhaps I'll come out of this with really long black fake eyelashes). This time, the fatigue is taking longer to dissipate, and when I look back on my first chemo, I can't recollect the body that managed to hike four or five miles just a week afterwards. It's a staggering fatigue. The body is heavy, especially the feet and the arms. There's the need, while lying down, to plot the efficient route before getting up—how, for example, to get the glass of water, the newspaper, the cup of green tea, the Advil and the cat onto the bed in one trip. The mind thickens. A week ago four wonderful books on Tibetan Buddhism arrived from Amazon. I was delighted to have them but had no actual memory of ordering them. The only explanation I could offer myself was that I had abused my credit card in a chemo brain black out. Fortunately, my friend Connie emailed me a day or so later warning me to look out for a package.

On top of this is paranoia about what the symptoms MEAN. Is my chemo brain worse than others? Is it "normal" to feel it more now that I have an impaired immune system? Is fatigue the beginning of the end or is fatigue a stage? Is there something people are not telling me? Is fatigue the same thing as a bad attitude? Why can't I sleep through the night, even with Ativan? How long does it take to get addicted? Are my eyelashes going? Will the vein in the crook of my left arm ever stop hurting? Why does the nausea last longer than it used to? Should I stop eating tomatoes, as both the oncologist and the herbologist recommend, even though when I crave food I crave tomatoes? Etcetera. Which is not to bitch and moan (though under the circumstances, it's been pointed out to me, I am bloody well entitled to complain) but to indicate that I tend to hover over myself in a way that I didn't before.

I observe myself as a living creature invaded by poisons that are supposed to exterminate the migrating cells of an enemy I cannot visualize: the electron microscope photograph of a cancer cell on the icebox? a new potato? a diffuse white gritty mass? I can only get better if I have the right attitude, which means hating cells that I cannot see. I am supposed to want more than anything else to destroy the little fuckers if they put an exploratory toe across the frontier of my body—never mind that I have no real knowledge of the little fuckers—because we know already that THEY, the little fucker cancer cells, are all by nature bad. Every last one must be removed from my body no matter how much it costs financially and physically because otherwise my body will fail under their weight, causing me terrible pain and my friends consternation and misery. Thanks to weed killer, the immune system that I need to fight the cancer cells is being sacrificed to the fight against the cancer cells. The medical profession finds fighting more attractive than figuring out how or why or where or whether to fight. It's all about purity and pollution. It's the language of the border police and of racists. It neither lowers my stress nor increases my strength to use such language. Doesn't hatred damage the one who hates more than the one who is hated?

The bitter irony of all this militarism is that it's yet another way to blame the victim. If I "lose" it means either that I didn't fight hard enough (80% of this is attitude, says my oncologist) or that I was so weak I succumbed to stress. Either way it's my problem, just as catching cancer supposedly was in the first place (bad breakup? too much administrative work? bad genes?). Forget about systematic industrial poisoning, drug company greed, and sexist, homophobic research protocols. If I win, I've "won" a battle defined in terms that mean I've lost just by not being a conscientious objector.

Other ways to think about this are hard to find and harder still to absorb. Learning to fight for yourself IS a way of reducing stress, the support group facilitator said to me recently. And there's the Dalai Lama. Pema Chodron. *The Tibetan Book of Living and Dying*. Ruth Remen's *Kitchen Table Wisdom*. All of these involve saying the words "someday I am going to die" rather than burying that fact, no pun intended. Detachment. Compassion. I can't do this all day, or every day. Instead, I gulp down cancer stories, like sugar, wherever I find them. I like the ones with the good endings. I search for the perfect narrative, meaning someone just like me, writing twenty years later about a memory. I skim the ones that are going to end badly, meaning too soon or in pain or in emotional disaster. I feel ripped off if what I think will be a good story turns out to be a bad one. I resent people who die with a good attitude.

Last chemo, my little sister Linda came and stayed for a week. She will come back after my final round next Thursday. She has been calling every two or three days since my diagnosis at the end of May, making it clear that she is willing to come to LA from Florida and stay as long as she is needed. She would have come earlier, but I had been saving her visit until I needed it. Also, I must say, I am afraid of visits from or with my family, even if the specific example of my family is my sister. My mother and I and a husband getting on to 70 are all the family Linda has. Our father is dead and so is our brother. My mother will soon be 77. I had dreaded actually asking Linda to do simple things. Before she came, I used to wake in the middle of the night in a panic about making small requests of her. I didn't want her to see me bald, or sick, or thin. I wanted to spare her. In truth, I wanted to spare myself. I did not want to depend, and I did not want to hear her say no or wait a minute if I got myself around to depending. Could I please have a glass of water? Could you please fluff the pillows? Could you please change the kitty litter?

It is hard to ask these things of your baby sister. Before Linda arrived, I worried out loud to my mother, except instead of confessing to my fear of humiliation I told her that I was worried about having to entertain Linda. In general, I don't confide in my mother, but this time I did. My mother told me not to be ridiculous. Linda knows she's there to help, she said. You don't have to entertain her. Linda came and watered and fluffed and changed and also washed dishes and did laundry and hiked down to the grocery store and screened telephone calls and pulled out the garbage cans, all with discretion and sensitivity and kindness. It took a heavy weight off Kim, who is trying to maintain a work schedule and her girlfriend too in a situation where I get the attention and she does the shit work. I still think of my little sister, especially when she purses her mouth to concentrate, as an innocent curly-haired little blonde thing, instead of a fifty-year-old woman trying to do yoga and preserve her own health.

Sweet serious Linda. Are you less afraid of me dying? I asked her. Yes, she replied, without hesitation. Are you? I had to think.

I'd always thought I would be the one to get something like this, Linda said one day while we were sitting on the sofa. You never got sick and I always had something or another. Then she looked at my feet and said, they're so small. We put our bare soles together so that she could prove her feet were bigger. I am glad she didn't catch breast cancer and I hope from the bottom of my heart that she never does, even though the fact of my catching it increases her chances, and my mother's, just like that.

Which is the only thing that happens just like that. When you have cancer, your world falls apart and then you realize that you can put it back together but you do not want it put back together in exactly the same way. This is one of the things Eve Sedgwick mentions in her remarkable *Dialogue on Love*, where breast cancer and bone metastasis play the background to a description of psychotherapy. Sedgwick was diagnosed at forty-one. She is thankful to be fifty. She doesn't have too much hair, or so it appears in the picture I study in *MAMM: Women, Cancer and Community*, and doesn't the existence of such a freebie make you want to bomb something?

Catching cancer is so shitty that you want utopia to spring from the rubble. You want life to mean something. You want to say what you have to say and you do not want other people to toy with the truth or with you or with their fears. You don't want to waste time. You don't want people to avoid the subject of death. You want to say everything you haven't said. You want to give away every possession you ever thought you cared about. You want to lavish gifts on everyone you know who gets cancer. You want wars and bombings and rape and torture and beatings and hatred and stupidity and greed to stop, just like that. You think about not killing ants and you wonder how Buddhists manage and then kill an ant or two anyway, for the fun of it, because you are angry and you have something to be angry about. You want to go back to the beginning and start with your family and remake it, but families change, if ever, at a glacial pace, and in my family there aren't many of us left to change. Still, I can see the iceberg cracking and perhaps Her Baldness is the beginning of the calving.

We talked about this last night in my support group, after the facilitator began the meeting by announcing the death of one woman who had been a member. I had never met her. No one else seemed to want to hear about her. I got the impression that no one would be going to the memorial service. Five women, two bald, one just growing back the fuzz, one with all her hair back just fine, talking about the mothers and fathers who failed them a long time ago trying hard to make it different this time round. Naomi is so depressed that the flesh on her face has softened and sagged and she has fantasies about doing bad things to other people with her kitchen knives. Better homicide than suicide, she jokes. Leslie, whose grandmother had breast cancer and whose mother was just diagnosed with the same thing, is afraid to take the genetic test she should take before her vacation. She doesn't want the results to mess up her plans. Glenda's mother died of cancer when Glenda was seven. Her father packed his four children off to the grandparents. Now Glenda has cancer and her youngest child is ten. You don't understand, Glenda says, what it's like not to have someone who would spin on a dime for you and do anything for you and listen to you and tell you they cared whenever you needed it. You're having a mother fantasy, we say. Real mothers are not like that. She doesn't believe us. She is redecorating her kids' rooms so that they can have memories, in case she might not be there. It's the way Glenda ends a lot of her sentences, delicately, looking down, ". . . in case I might not be there." Louanne isn't at group. Rumor has it that she has missed another chemo appointment.

Thus supported, Her Baldness sails back from Santa Monica to Silver Lake, all clear with the exception of one minor looky loo on the left lane of the 110, past the Staples Center and the Democratic Convention and the giant video projections of Al Gore and weird red white and blue streamers coming off the tops of buildings and skyscrapers bathed in light that's also supposed to be red white and blue but somehow looks a little too rainbow. One of our tribe must have graduated to exterior decoration. Somewhere below the freeway the storm troopers are shooting rubber bullets and people are moving much faster than Her Baldness, who is operating at a different speed and is, as a result, missing the whole drama. She has a sore scalp and her black cap needs washing. She thinks people haven't exactly been giving her the straight story and that she'll be lucky if she has some fine down by November. She speculates that as her hair did not fall out all at once so it will not grow back in all at once. What's on her scalp looks like a combination of five o' clock shadow and infant fuzz. Her armpit hair is thin to nonexistent, and the same is true of her pubic hair, but fortunately her girlfriend is more than a bit of a pervert. The eyebrows are still there but the eyelashes are itchy.

THURSDAY | AUGUST 17, 2000

Blood count up to 3,800. Meet Dr. Palmer, the radiation oncologist. Nutritionist is called in to explain how to maintain weight. Watch out for burn and fatigue, says Dr. P.

Kim returns from an overnight to Miami. She wants air conditioning. I protest. We need to be more conscious about energy conservation, I tell her. We can just move more slowly. We'll get used to hot air. I live here too! she screams. It's not fair!

IN A MESSAGE DATED
8/17/00 CBLORD@UCI.EDU
WRITES TO FOCL'SRB:

SUBJECT: SHARI HATT'S FOUR BATH SEQUENCE FOR HEAVY
DETOX

1. 10 baths
   2 lbs. baking soda
   30 mins.
   Submerge hands

2. 10 baths
   3 pints hydrogen peroxide
   Submerge hands

3. 6 baths
   $1/2$ box borax
   20 minutes
   Submerge hands

4. 6 baths
   $1/2$ box borax
   2 pints hydrogen peroxide
   20 minutes
   Submerge hands

FRIDAY | AUGUST 18, 2000

IN A MESSAGE DATED
8/18/00 JANECO WRITES:

Victoria, a character on *One Life to Live*, has spent about a month of weekly episodes dealing with cancer. Her husband to be #8 probably was very supportive as were her two adult male children. They said love and had group hugs so often that I began to feel very ill. Just before she was declared cancer free she went to see her evil ex father-in-law. She wanted to show him something. She removed her wig which was very expensive cos it didnt look like a wig and revealed a bald head. It was very tanned perhaps this was an added tanning treatment that she got with chemo.

Thank god, america and McDonalds for soap operas that enlighten us all.

In the immortal words of Nurse Katie, purveyor of chemicals, Joan is "no longer a chemo virgin."

SUBJECT: RECENT ACCESSIONS, COLLECTION OF HER BALDNESS, DEPARTMENT OF ACRONYMS

PWC	Person With Cancer
PBGO	Person Barely Getting Over
BBP	Bald Barfing Person
WAPHMO	Woman About to Go Postal at HMO
PSHIFTY	Person Still Hanging in Fine Thank You
QIBIFA	Quite Ill But, Inexplicably, Fat Anyway
WOBT	Woman on Borrowed Time

Courtesy Eve Kosofsky Sedgwick,
MAMM (23:2), handed out at the support group

SATURDAY | AUGUST 19, 2000

you can pretty much count on this truth: if a teacher is really important to a student, the reverse will also be true. and also i must confess i loved your dimples from the getgo.

I do believe in reincarnation. It's the only story that makes sense to me.

And Alexandra David-Neel has some beautiful descriptions of Mahayana Buddhist physics. Her version of reincarnation is not about a "me" or "ego" continuing on, but a self (in a poststructuralist way) as a crossroads of fragments of many selves, kind of magnetized together for some period of time. They can be from a myriad of places and times. They surface and then dive again. So we're all these bundles of lives passing each other, participating in this kind of organization of matter. We are not that different from the "things" and "spaces" we inhabit.

Damn the oncologists saying "80% of this is attitude". As though they themselves have nothing to do with it. I think one possible basic reality of all this is that the PWBrCa has very little control, so shouldn't waste precious energy worrying about exercising it over a realm that has a life of its own, narrowing and widening, from the body to the abyss and back again. Did you read in the *Times* that whining is now considered a good thing?

IN A MESSAGE DATED
8/19/00 VOLT WRITES:
Your pals are right, you should have cut it sooner.

IN A MESSAGE DATED
8/19/00 CBLORD@UCI.EDU
WRITES TO UNDISCLOSED
RECIPIENTS:
SUBJECT: HER BALDNESS STARTS A RUMOR

Lorraine O'Grady, way back at the beginning of August, before chemo number three, started it. Her Baldness had been bitching and moaning. have you seen any black lesbians lately? Lorraine asked. And also, would bald read differently in Dominica?

So, sheepish about not being bald, black or proud, and not, in sad fact, having lately seen in passing or answered the door to anyone of the BBP description, I put myself in my place and decided to tackle the Dominica question. If I could skip the rest of chemo and radiation too and beam myself to Dominica tomorrow, instead of taking the redeye to San Juan and then a puddle jumper, this is what it would look like. Her Baldness rents her mouldy Suzuki on Bath Road and drives to the bay front. She goes to the ATM at the Royal Bank of Canada for Eastern Caribbean dollars, then Coco Rico for bread and cheese and then Whitchurch's round the corner for a few staples.

Just thinking about the sun makes my scalp burn, and even if I change the scene to the cool of the morning or after a rain shower, I can't get to Dominica from here. There is no community of shaved black men, shaved white men, shaved gay men, or shaved bald black and proud lesbians or shaved bald white and proud lesbians into which Chemo Girl could blend. In Dominica the choice is between dreads and combovers. Her Baldness would be on her own.

Cancer hasn't, however, spared the so-called nature island, where the off-shore banks are breeding faster than crapaud. I needed information and so I started, as I often do, with the Honychurch family. Patricia, now in her mid-seventies, was a friend of my parents. Her son Lennox, born a few weeks after my brother Robert in the old Roseau hospital, is the island's unofficial historian. When Lennox received his D. Phil from Oxford a few years ago, the banner headline in *The Chronicle* read DOCTOR LENNOX!!!!! The story, with photographs, took up the entire front page, except for a little filler item titled, MAN EATS BULB, but that was about another man, someone in Wesley or Marigot, as I recall. Just to put in perspective the importance of the Honychurch name in Dominica, as it may not be evident to those of you who live in the rest of the world, there is a story told about a tourist who went to get a bite to eat at the Fort Young Hotel, where Lennox was lunching with Mick Jagger. (Dominica is one of the places where the rich and famous come to hide.) "Is that Mick Jagger?" asked the incredulous tourist. "No," said the waiter, impatiently. "Everyone knows that's Lennox Honychurch." This is a true story.

I often rent Patricia's cottage, and when I do I take meals with her and with her daughter and her grandchildren. Patricia is extremely kind to me, and we are quite fond of each other. Sometime in July, I emailed Patricia. Are chemo and radiation available at the Princess Margaret Hospital? Patricia didn't know, but she got me the email address of a doctor I could ask, and made the cyber introductions. She also telephoned her half sister Daphne, now in her mid-eighties and indisputably the grande dame of all the white settlers, to relay my questions. My friend John Mason Kirby arrived at the beginning of August to check on the fields of anthuriums he had recently planted with the help of Marie Theophile up at Castleton on the Imperial Road where the handpainted sign at the bottom of the driveway still says NO TRESSPASSING with a total of four Ss because Moyda Kelly who came there with her husband Charles after she had fled the Nazis did not like uninvited visitors and would chase them off the property screaming obscenities of such linguistic inventiveness than only the occasional German or Austrian tourist could really apprehend their venom. By the time John arrived, or so he emailed me, EVERYONE was really worried that I would try to come to Dominica for chemo and radiation.

Daphne took upon herself the responsibility of writing me a proper letter to stop me from any such foolishness. She mailed her letter on

August 6, right after she got wind of my questions, but the Silver Lake post office being worse than the Roseau post office, I didn't receive Daphne's letter for two weeks, that is, just a few days ago. Daphne reminds me that the longstanding joke about the Princess Margaret Hospital is that you have to be very strong and well to survive it. She asks me why I suppose people go the great United States—there would be a slow sarcasm in the way she pronounced those last three words—to get treatment for anything serious. She adds that cancer is a serious thing and advises me, in no uncertain terms, to stay where I am lucky enough to be.

In the meantime, before Daphne's letter arrived, I emailed and wrote everyone concerned, apologizing for any misunderstanding that might have been caused by my hypothetical questions about what would have happened to me had I been living my parallel life. (In which case, however, the questions would probably have been moot because I would not have been exposed to such stress factors as electricity, bitter ex lovers, stressful administrative jobs or allegedly incomprehensible critical theory involving sexuality.) I reassured Patricia that I planned to finish my chemo, do radiation, and rebuild my immune system in Los Angeles, where, as Patricia politely said in the first place, I am surely better off.

According to Dr. Natashia Grell Aird, breast and cervical cancer are the most common cancers in Dominica. There is a competent general surgeon who can do the necessary in the way of mastectomies, radical mastectomies and modified radical mastectomies. There are facilities for mammogram screening, and there is a radiologist to read the mammograms. However, there is neither an oncologist nor facilities for radiation or chemo, though Tamoxifen, which can be administered orally, is a possibility. Dominicans who need chemo or radiation are referred to Martinique, Guadeloupe, or Barbados. Some people have insurance that covers them. Those who have neither insurance nor money do not receive treatment. There may well be bush remedies for cancer, says Dr. Aird, but she reminds me that no such remedies have been proven effective.

It would be extremely unusual, says Dr. Aird, for a woman not to cover her baldness in any way.

This is not just because bald is not a practical costume in strong sun or because hair and hair extenders (manufactured in Taiwan) are powerful signifiers in Dominica. Due to the complete lack of facilities for treatment, baldness resulting from infusions of weed killer wouldn't be a legible sign in Roseau. Her Baldness would not signify the idea of chemo as a transitory state of affairs. Her Baldness, strolling down the bay front in the cool of the day, would read as a sick old woman coming to Dominica to spend her last days in what she had been led to believe was paradise. Because she is thin, Her Baldness could well read as someone with an AIDS-related illness, which is shorthand for homo, that is to say an import, as distinguished from zami or mako or man royal or tanti man, of which there are plenty but they are not homo, and in Dominica it is homos, not the particular sexual acts of makos or zamis, who are the cause of AIDS. The practices of homos are illegal in Dominica under the recently renewed Sexual Offenders Act.

Her Baldness would be a topic of public discussion. She might achieve *The Chronicle*, which prints pictures of people with AIDS on the front page, to say nothing of fetuses left in the gutters of Roseau. Her Baldness would be a freak, that's what she's trying to say. She feels like a freak in Los Angeles, though she does her best to be a bold freak, and she'd feel like more of a freak in Dominica, where baldness would make her whiter and sick too, where baldness would be a nakedness akin to the wearing of short shorts or bathing suits on the streets of Roseau. Too, there's not much sense in Dominica of serious illness as a curable event, and the timing of Her Baldness's departure from this world would be discussed with more of a sense of imminence than it is here in Los Angeles, as far as I know.

SUNDAY | AUGUST 20, 2000

IN A MESSAGE DATED 8/20/00 CBLORD@UCI.EDU WRITES TO JEANNIES:

the basic idea is that i should eat a lot, so i will start with the two apple pies you left us.

IN A MESSAGE DATED
8/20/00 SRANKAIT WRITES: Most of us, myself included, learned how to wait and may be (somewhat) good at waiting things out (sometimes) but even with "chemo brain" you are connecting so vividly with life. I always see myself as being like the dog or cat that goes into the basket or off to some remote part of the lawn to either heal or try to go with some grace (talk about romantic self deception). In reading what you wrote today I feel like a real coward.

Kim and I head for a weekend fling at Shutters. We have always meant to splurge on a night there. The valet asks about our luggage. I thought YOU put it in the trunk, we say to each other. We realize we have left it on the street in front of our house. We squabble. We call Annie. She rescues it. By the time we have driven across town and back again to Santa Monica, we have been upgraded to the only remaining room, the presidential suite: living room, bedroom, two bathrooms, kitchen, two fireplaces, ocean view, orgy-sized jacuzzi. Brad and Jennifer, it is whispered, departed only a few days ago. Tears, butterfly sex, tears, dinner in front of the fireplace. The service is impeccable. We might be important, not just two ordinary middle-aged lesbians scared out of their minds. I don't know my body. I can't find its pleasure. It's not safe to let it out. It's not safe to look. It is not safe to try to see into the future. I watch people in the wet wide low tide between land and sea, softening their gait, feeling the sand on their bare feet, standing up to their ankles in water, chattering, caressing, hopping—behaving like all creatures that breathe air at the limit of their world. I try to fill my lungs but can't. My chest isn't big enough to hold the dread. Reading about being in the moment is not the same as being in the moment. Wanting not to fear death isn't the same as not fearing death.

Peggy calls. If I had had no treatment whatsoever, breast cancer would have killed me in a year or so. I have a 5% chance of recurrence in my right breast. The chances in my left breast are the same as for any other woman. When a treatment gives only a 1 to 3% improvement in statistical probability, doctors seldom want to do it. Patients almost always do. Of course I can travel in November. Radiation is nothing.

I am beginning to say, more often, JUST ONE MORE.

MONDAY | AUGUST 21, 2000

IN A MESSAGE DATED
8/21/00 CBLORD@UCI.EDU
WRITES TO VOLT: it's very hard for me actually to feel loved, especially in this fragile moment when i turn to water and it all pours out my eyes. we have tickets to paris, which, as we don't live there, it seems fabulous and

romantic and beautiful, arriving dec 21 and leaving dec 27. are you around? can you be?

My department chair calls. The dean wants to know whether the new assistant professor can have my office. Tacky. No.

TUESDAY | AUGUST 22, 2000

Is the shrink trying to cheer me up?

WEDNESDAY | AUGUST 23, 2000

Kim is overwhelmed. Kim is drowning in fear. Kim doesn't want Paris. Kim wants to be with family at Christmas. What family? Her mother hasn't managed to send us a card. Her mother thinks I should go to chemo by myself. I need a blockbuster trip. I want Kim with me in a wholehearted way. Plan the trip, even if you have to cancel, says the shrink, who gives me a good big hug on my way out the door.

IN A MESSAGE DATED 8/23/00 CBLORD@UCI.EDU WRITES TO FOCL'SRB:

SUBJECT: SELECTED ACCESSIONS, MISC., COLLECTION OF HER BALDNESS

Her Baldness acknowledges the following, with gratitude:

Black billed cap with SUPREME and eight stars embroidered in yellow and gray

Paul Cox's *Nafanua*

La Bastide soap and salts and bubbles

A subscription to *Yoga Journal* and a London bus key ring

Taxco bracelet and ring

Scanned and enlarged postage stamp (UK) of Captain Cook with a bald tattooed man

Windup tin photographer and Zadie Smith's *White Teeth*

Audio tapes of the last Harry Potter book

Tom Brokaw, *The Greatest Generation* (Reader's Digest large type edition) and Dava Sobel, *Galileo's Daughter*

Red bedside thermos with spigot

Rainbow key ring with added tag reading WORLD'S GREATEST THINKER

Several loaves of Boulud bakery bread

One pair Target bedroom slippers, pale blue and glitter shag

Four books on Tibetan Buddhism

One organic tomato

Two page typed MS of story about a lesbian lady teacher

Sacred Mirrors: The Visionary Art of Alex Grey

Christopher Brookmyre, assorted Scottish noir mysteries

Gray plaster dog Buddha in meditation pose

Large gift basket with pillow, throw, bath oil, and candle

Summer issues of *The Dominica Chronicle*

One moose paperweight and approximately one dozen plastic bracelets in the shape of barbed wire

Patrick O'Brian paperbacks

Various pictures of Kofi and Rio

One stone from Macchu Picchu

THURSDAY | AUGUST 24, 2000

Deborah calls. Watch out for depression once you're finished. And anger.

Linda calls.

Betty calls.

IN A MESSAGE DATED
8/24/00 CBLORD@UCI.EDU
WRITES TO UNDISCLOSED
RECIPIENTS: SUBJECT: HER BALDNESS GETS A LESSON IN PHOTOGRAPHY
My studio is a mess. I hate putting things away. Every surface is piled
with xeroxes and books and slides because I hate putting things away.
I'm not much good at self promotion, and I don't like the shit work
entailed in seeing to one's own history. (In this as in other ways, I feel
like I have failed as a feminist, but that's another story.) BrCa, however,
has seemed a sufficiently important event in my life to document it.
Also, I think of breast cancer as finite and therefore manageable. Writing about breast cancer and photographing myself with breast cancer
is not something I plan to do for the rest of my life. It's something I am
doing now, because later I won't remember every detail and because I
won't want to remember every detail. In addition, I've needed to make
for myself a little community of people, if not all in physical presence—
since so many of HB's readers do not live in Los Angeles—at least people
who have in one very real way or another been here for me with calls
and gifts and love and rides, people who read their email.

The documentation jones has led me to photograph the dismal moments—the head shaving, the syringes and tubes, the uplifting cheerful art in the doctors' offices, the doctors, the blood count machine,
the soaking in baking soda baths, the lying around in bed and so forth.
Kim helps. We use the point-and-shoot that she gave me for our second
Christmas. Folks in the oncologist's office are getting used to the flash
going off. I say, frame that, take that, tilt it up or tilt it down, and Kim

does the actual button pushing. It's frustrating not to be the person behind the camera and see what's inside the rectangle. A wiser and more patient woman might have saved up the rolls of film until the hair and the color and the energy were back. Not me. Last week I picked up in Larchmont a few packets of photomat prints, in duplicate. I must have expected that will and accessories would triumph over weed killer and an on-camera flash.

Not so. I look like a bad Nicholas Nixon photo of an AIDS victim, I wail to Kim on the phone, except that I don't have Kaposi's. Why didn't you tell me? Why did you let me go out of the house? You DON'T look terrible, said Kim, ever reasonable, ever loving. Photography lies. Put them away until you're better.

But I'm a sunburn peeler and fingernail biter and scab picker and I know the real trouble with photography is that it only lies most of the time. I hated Nicholas Nixon for making victim photos and now here I am doing it to myself, setting it up so that I hold in my hands myself going from a pink cheeked mischievous woman with her new dyke short haircut standing in the bathroom dressed in a ragged 58% DON'T WANT PERSHINGS T-shirt and trying to shave her own head to a bald depressed woman sitting on an iron bedstead covering her nakedness with a bath towel to a woman in a white cap sticking her over-accessorized arm out for a red drip in the oncologist's office to a woman in a black cap with her feet tucked up on a chair, looking smaller than she remembers, to a woman who has stripped off her black cap because she is having one of the unbelievably intense hot flashes that result from chemo because chemo destroys the reproductive system to a naked bald woman in a bathtub.

I am setting myself up. The face gets thinner. The shadows under the eyes darken. Chemo stains. In some of the photographs I am yellow and in some I am dead white. Muscles don't hold the bones up in quite the same way. I look like someone who's trying but can't quite manage, three months after the beginning of the BrCa experience, to keep it together. It's a fine distinction, I admit, but the photographs don't seem to me as much self-destructive as an insane act of aggression perpetrated by myself against myself. Some other me, the anthropologist or the pathologist or the evil scientist or the soldier, pointed the camera and snapped. It's all very well to say things like, "Go with the flow" or "The gift of cancer is that it teaches you you're not in control," but I have absolutely no power in these photographs, and the wrenching thing is that I took the power away from myself. I overhear Kim telling people on the phone that I am spinning into depression because I got back photographs and they were really unflattering. Unflattering is not the word. I look far worse than I want to feel or than I believe I look even when I'm turning everything I can muster, including my accessories, to the end of looking as good as possible. Good here means alive. But will alone does not a positive image make. I don't buy the whole positive image school of thought but I had the arrogance to think I was smarter than my camera and it turns out not to be so. I do not want to face myself sick.

The impulse behind these photographs exists in a grammatical space I don't yet inhabit. I make them because I want to have them when I inhabit a tense I have not yet lived to see. I want to use them as blocks in a language that I should like the opportunity to learn. These are the sentences I want to say, one of these days. I look like shit in these pictures, but I took them when I used to have breast cancer. I took them when I had breast cancer. I took them when I once had breast cancer, and that was a long summer. I don't want the photographs to become elements of someone else's third person pluperfect: that was the summer Catherine had breast cancer, that was the summer she began to go downhill, that was the summer she would have finished her book.

Hannah Wilke, whose *Intra-Venus* I love and have often taught as a demonstration of feminist agency and wicked wit, hadn't intended a documentation of her death by lymphoma, much less a documentation of her own courage. She set out to record her return from the descent. She wanted to be in your face with her body because her body was the medium to which she was always returned and so she made it the medium which she got to first. I unshuffle the sequence of photo-

graphs to tell the story I now understand in finer detail: a slim silhou-
ette in the shower, before the chemo made her put on a lot of weight
(yes, this happens); the incision at the lymph nodes in her neck; the
thin long tresses, wet in the shower; the short fuzz; the shaved pate and
the defiant tilt of the chin; the disappearing pubic hair; the gorgeous
silky white femme lingerie, no matter what; the clowning and posing
with the hospital props which are, after all, the only toys you have when
they take your stuff away and make you wait and wait for the next medical event. If I run the movie backwards in my head, I can give Hannah
a happy ending: downy new hair, circles under the eyes fading, color
flushing her cheeks, weight returning to normal, the cleansing showers as the fatigue lifts, the energy filling her face. Cured. That was the
title Wilke had in mind.

I've kept a tally of cases worse than mine. I've already confessed to this.
It's not just tacky to do this, it's SICK, far from Buddhism of any kind,
worse than feeling competitive about your triangle in a yoga class, and
an infantile way to deal with issues of mortality, but there it is. Here's
my file. A man with breast cancer. The sort of breast cancer that shows
up in the lymph nodes but can't be located anywhere in the breasts
("the unknown primary"). The sort of breast cancer that does not appear on x rays, even though a lump is palpable. A surgical wound that
can heal only by "primary intention." If such a wound is stitched up an
infection begins, so the open hole in the body is bandaged and left to
heal, on its own. Sometimes this sort of wound has to be washed and
rebandaged daily. I cannot imagine anything more terrifying than looking through a hole directly into the interior of my body, but the thing
which actually haunts me more than the image of the interior of my
body is the idea that the body can repair such a wound.

Last chemo is today at 2 p.m. THE LAST CHEMO. Everyone says this
to me with the same inflection: Catherine, it's the LAST chemo. It's a
good day. I will keep the rock from Macchu Picchu with me, because
it's a place I will go one day, along with a pumice pebble from the side
of the Boiling Lake in Dominica. Kim and I will keep photographing
because just like the chemo, it's too late to stop. Kim will stay with me

on Friday and for the weekend. Annie is flying down from San Francisco on Monday, and Linda is coming on Tuesday for a week. Ativan is on hand. Phone calls are welcome. Her Baldness isn't doing this on her own.

TUESDAY | AUGUST 29, 2000

IN A MESSAGE DATED 8/29/00 ANNEJUN WRITES: your sister's a really beautiful woman. i wish i had that kind of roundness. ain't it always better on someone else's lawn?

WEDNESDAY | AUGUST 30, 2000

IN A MESSAGE DATED 8/30/00 JEANNIES WRITES: i'm around and happy to help out or stop by or change the cat litter or rent a movie or read to you in bed or water the plants or just call or whatever.

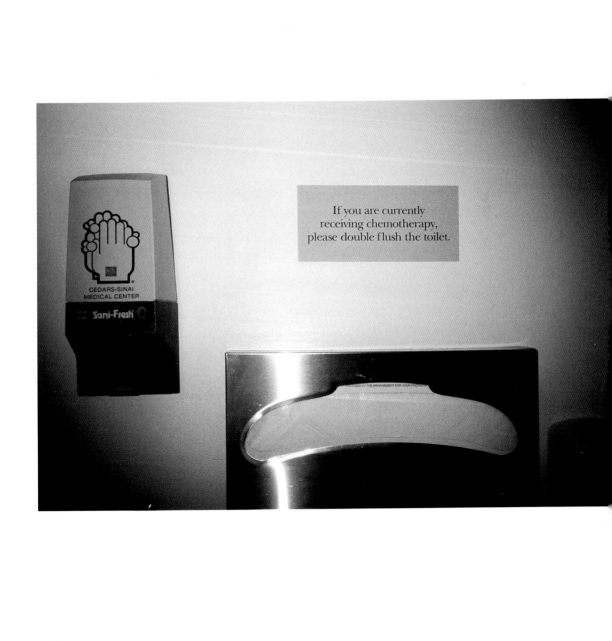

SEPTEMBER | 2000

FRIDAY | SEPTEMBER 1, 2000

Group. Louanne goes after the facilitator who loses it with her then comes back to remind us that this is a room of healing and we are trying to help. Perhaps I have something to learn about teaching.

SUNDAY | SEPTEMBER 3, 2000

I would rather be alive than have my hair, no matter if it comes back uneven and sparse. The lump in my right breast is bigger than ever.

MONDAY | SEPTEMBER 4, 2000

Insomnia. Twinges. Lumps. Ticking. Kim is having a horrible time at work. We take a twenty-minute walk in the a.m. I can barely keep up.

TUESDAY | SEPTEMBER 5, 2000

IN A MESSAGE DATED 9/5/00 AVEST WRITES: Do we wait five years, or is there another intervention to come?

WEDNESDAY | SEPTEMBER 6, 2000

IN A MESSAGE DATED 9/6/00 MGEVE WRITES: The shampoo and gel are delicious, just the thing for a stressed out, depressed sweatshop worker who wishes she had done adjunct classes in NY instead of walking into a rat's nest of disorganized, contentious pettiness. Going home for the weekend. Hooray, though this means that I won't be there if you and Kim go on the 24th. We'll hook up another time, I'm sure and hope in the meantime your strength is coming back and life looks a little rosier. Will call when I'm not in such a bad mood.

Wee baby moon at 5 a.m. My sister has only one friend where she lives, and she cannot talk to her freely because her politics are so conservative. Don't, Kim says. Linda is happy with her life. And this time Linda is more relaxed, content to be wined and dined. Last night's celebration dinner too rich for me, Kim too tired to love it, but Linda closed her eyes, put a little bit on the end of her tongue and licked like a kitten. We need to live closer, says Kim, putting into words what the WASP sisters don't. Linda gets on the Super Shuttle with a bulging suitcase and new black shirt. We both weep.

IN A MESSAGE DATED 9/6/00 CBLORD@UCI.EDU WRITES TO UNDISCLOSED RECIPIENTS:

SUBJECT: COLLECTION OF HER BALDNESS, DEPARTMENT OF PERSPECTIVE

We would like to think that early detection is the answer, and it is . . . for some women. But most breast cancers are present for eight to ten years by the time they can be felt or seen on a mammogram. The breast cancer cells have the ability to get out of the breast into the blood vessels very early, at about year one or two. From there they can spread throughout the body, and they do. Whether they persist depends on their ability to survive in another organ as well as on the immune system's ability to destroy them. Studies have shown that regular screening mammography can find cancer at a curable stage in 30 percent of women over the age of fifty. That is a lot . . . But it is only 30 percent, not 100 percent. That is because some cancers are so slow growing that they will never spread. Others are so fast growing that they have spread by the time we have found them. Many women will have their cancers detected by mammography and still die of the disease. Breast self-exam is even less successful at making a difference in breast cancer survival. SUSAN LOVE, introduction to Hollis Sigler, *Breast Cancer Journal* (1999)

The paradox in cancer is that although each cancer is a clone, it is the *lack* of genetic uniformity that is the key to its imperialistic success. Cancer clones evolve and diversify, over variable but usually very protracted periods of years and decades, by sequential addition of mutations in different genes that collectively corrupt cell behaviour. These then provide a genetic passport through the major evolutionary bottlenecks: the initial formation of a tumour; next, tumour to cancer transition with spread within tissues followed by dissemination or metastasis to other tissues; and then, finally, survival of the decimation elicited by therapy . . . The winning cellular phenotypes are very rare, the drop-out rate is huge, but the culmination of this process is a mutinous species of cell or clone that has shut off the safety valves of differentiation and death, and reproduces itself continually as an immortal clone with territorial dominance of the body habitat.   MEL GREAVES, *Cancer: The Evolutionary Legacy* (2000)

THURSDAY | SEPTEMBER 7, 2000

Lynn B. calls. You don't deserve it. No one does, but you really don't.

FRIDAY | SEPTEMBER 8, 2000

Group. A little rebellion against the facilitator. We resist her plans to spend half an hour reading the schedule of yoga and art therapy and meditation for the entire month ahead. We want to talk to each other. Geraldine is the only one who has never taken off her wig in public. It slipped while she was shopping yesterday. She is distraught.

The thing about cancer is that your ex-lovers want to visit.

SATURDAY | SEPTEMBER 9, 2000

IN A MESSAGE DATED 9/9/00 CBLORD@UCI.EDU WRITES TO FOCL'SRB:

SUBJECT: HER BALDNESS GRADUATES

Women who do chemo name them by numbers the way lab technicians name their mice or bureaucrats name streets. You don't want to squander too much imagination on the naming. Chemo Number One, that was ok, Chemo Number Two, it got worse, Chemo Number Three, not too bad, though that very morning my (former) accountant called to say she had lost all my tax information for my already late 1999 returns, and, Chemo Number Four, also not too bad, even though the hot water heater blew up a few days later.

Women who do chemo remember the exact date of each and every one. June 20, July 13, August 3, August 24. Those are mine. Perhaps the dates will fade one day into a generality such as "July and August of 2000" or the even more splendidly abstract "summer of 2000," but right now there are four chemos and they are distinct. Chemo Number Four was not, in fact, too bad. Beforehand I sat cross legged in the living room to meditate, something that in sad fact I don't often achieve. I faced the window and shut my eyes and then recalled that the idea is not to shut one's eyes but to keep them open without bringing the attention to what might be seen. The morning light picked a single leaf out of the Chinese elm that makes shade over our back deck, causing a tiny green specificity to float in front of a mass of shadow. Everything seemed, at that exact moment, entirely well with me and with my world. I called to mind the people who have loved me through this. I turned the image of each and every one of them around and about in my head. This was even better than the leaf. I made a list of places I want to get to: the Haida villages, Borobudur, the dolmens of Brittany, Macchu Picchu, the rock drawings of Northern Australia and Horseshoe Canyon in Utah.

Then David interrupted his writing to come and pick me up, just as he did for Chemo Number Two. He was precisely on time, as he always is, and on the way to Cedars we stopped at the travel bookstore. I bought guide books to Paris and to Andalusia, where Kim and I are planning to celebrate at Christmas, so that there would be something to read and laugh about during the drip itself, absurd as the idea of planning such a trip may sound. Or planning. I also brought with me two undistinguished looking rocks. I laid them among the syringes and tubes. It helped, particularly by the end of the procedure, to hold tightly to a featherweight piece of white pumice from an obscure island and remind myself that the Boiling Lake is a legendarily difficult hike and that on my second trip there, after I tore the ligament in my ankle at the start of the trail back, I made it up and down three steep clay ridges on one leg and a stick. It helped, also, to see the relief on Kim's face when Chemo Number Four was over. It helped to learn, from Michelle the nurse, that NOBODY goes alone to chemo. It helped to get, just as the last syringe was finishing up, a certificate with fancy borders and a gold seal.

CONGRATULATIONS
Catherine Lord
You have successfully completed chemotherapy
We are so proud of you!
August 24, 2000
Michael Van Scoy Mosher, M.D. Michelle Wellisch, R.N.

And of course it helped that Kim stuck close for Friday and for the entire weekend, and that Annie came to visit on Monday while I reclined in bed. This is the hardest thing I've ever done, I said to her when we said goodbye. It was meant as a self-conscious bit of hyberbole to deflect attention from my tears, but as the words came out of my mouth, I realized they were true.

The thing about chemo is that you don't know whether it worked unless you learn down the road that it has failed. No news is good news. Susan Love says that one third of all women diagnosed with breast cancer will die. The odds of recovery have remained unchanged despite medical discoveries. Surgery alone cures about 70% of cancers. This is what Dr. Van Scoy Mosher says, putting a better face on things. I call him Michael because his name is so long (Michelle says that in the seventies he took his wife's name) and because he is, or once was, a friend of my doctor friends. My familiarity seems to annoy him slightly unless I am weeping, in which case I am excused. The thing about chemo, the truly SICK and most upsetting thing, is that after it's over, after you're back to normal, meaning a reduced schedule of meals and movies and friends, you spin out wondering whether you've suffered enough. Perhaps the last two doses were too light. Perhaps they measured the weed killer wrong. Perhaps if it hurt more, perhaps if I had done six chemos, or eight, instead of a dilettantish four, or gone on Taxol on my own volition, or perhaps the $5,000 a pop for Taxol was more than my oncologist thought I was worth, or perhaps if they had prescribed Tamoxifen, which Michael won't because I am estrogen receptor negative, perhaps then the cancer wouldn't come back.

I have more than a few nights in a row when such thoughts wake me. In turn, I wake Kim, who has agreed to sing me the following lullaby anywhere at any hour. I have taken her up on this offer all summer long and she has always been gracious about my requests.

There's a wee baby moon lying on her back
With her little silvery toes in the air
She's all by herself in the wide blue sky
But the little baby moon doesn't care

What you are feeling is perfectly common, Michael assures me, as I sit weeping on his hard blue sofa looking at his blackboard upon which he has made a crude drawing of infiltrating ductal carcinoma for the woman who was there before me. You have done everything you could, he says. The fear is normal. It will be even worse after radiation stops. It is normal to grow another lump exactly where the old one was. It's scar tissue. Lots of women get these lumps. Don't worry.

You get through chemo by investing the chemicals with power, Dr. Deena Nelson says, when I call her. She is an internist who specializes in cancer. She and her girlfriend, Dr. Peggy Kemeny, a surgeon who also specializes in cancer, live in New York. That they are friends who answer our questions honestly has been an enormous help to us. Once you've given the chemicals that power, you're bereft when you're not doing it any more, Deena says.

I feel absolutely alone in the wide blue sky.

Chemo is over. To celebrate I've thrown out the left over anti-barf Kytril, even if it cost fifty five U.S. dollars for ONE pill, the free samples of Zofran, the nonabrasive toothpaste and the booklets on "Oral Hygiene During Chemotherapy."

Is there life after chemo?

Julia Marie came to give me a massage. She works on my belly and neck. She has the touch of a child molester, so subtle it could always be denied. Her fingers walk into my ears. I accede. About halfway through it came to mind that I have also been meaning to climb Diablotin, the tallest mountain in Dominica at just over 5,000 feet, named for the trusting black-capped petrel that the greedy French used to bag from their nesting holes in such numbers that by the seventeenth century they were thought to be as dead as the dodo.

I went shopping with Linda, on her second visit of dishwashing and plant watering and cat feeding and general care taking. After I incited Linda to spend a lot of money on clothes one morning, $500 in an hour, we went to Out of the Closet, where I bought a jacket and pajama bottoms for seven dollars. The woman at the register, who had a distinct limp, took my money and asked if I was going through chemo. Yes. This gave her the opening to tell me about her experience with BrCa: two years ago, stage one, node-negative, now metastasized to her bones. Bad HMO or a bigger club than I want it to be? Why did she tell you this? Michael says in frustration when I phone him. It's like telling the person in line for a plane that your sister died in a crash last year. Why do you ask me these questions? he said in equal frustration when I asked him a few weeks ago how long I would have lived had I opted to forego surgery and chemo and radiation. A year or two, he replied, and it would not have been pretty.

And then there's the monitoring. When I went for the mammo that falls between Chemo Number Four and Radiation Number One (there will be either Thirty Three or Thirty Five, this is yet to be decided, but at any rate, for all practical purposes, it's five days a week for seven weeks — like psychoanalysis, says Yvonne) I did not have to wait in the waiting room. I am whisked out. Am I bad for client morale in my obvious eggheadedness beneath my little black cap? The waiting room into which I was ushered was larger than the one I was assigned for my routine screening last May. The pile of salmon smocks was likewise larger. The better to contemplate my mortality, there was a full-length mirror. I've spent a lot of time this summer considering enormous philosophical issues in rooms that are too small, too cold, too bright, have dark stain-concealing carpets, and involve formica. Either their walls are covered with small patterned wallpaper or they are painted salmon. They feature posters gone magenta of paintings by artists no one minds. Desktop stress-reducing fountains are also popular. The magazine selections are unsatisfying.

There was a new technician running the mammo machine, not Carlaloyce but an Indian woman who wore no name tag and found lumps left and right. She sent me a few doors down for an ultrasound, which was done by the same Natasha who discovered in May that the lump with irregular margins that might conceivably have been a fluid-filled cyst was in fact solid and abnormal. Natasha didn't remember me. Not only am I bald now but Natasha finds at least one cancer a day, and so there have been, since my particular 1.5 centimeters at 12 o'clock in the RBr, at least a hundred others. When I told Natasha that I remembered her, she was proud that she was the one to confirm my lump meant trouble. Her grandmother died twenty years ago in Russia. They didn't do mammograms in Russia then. It was too late by the time her grandmother found her lump. Presumably that's why Natasha spends her days in a windowless room slathering goop on tits. She keeps a chocolate box with a picture of Nefertiti between her diplomas above the light box. If everything's OK on the ultrasound, you see round black dots with regular margins, rather like those John Baldessari works from the eighties, floating above a white column. There were a great many black dots on my TV screen, but all of them floated above white columns. The techs, all women, congratulated me. I had gotten the card to a club I didn't know existed, the premiere executive automatic upgrade warm chocolate chip cookies first class seats on Air Cancer.

Her Baldness's pate now looks like the front part of Allan Sekula's head, which, as I am a little taller than Allan, I observed in some detail during a conversation we had at an opening on Friday night at the Korean American Museum. There's not much in the way of actual sprouts per square inch, but rather a very sparse covering perhaps a quarter of an inch long. I had thought that hair would return in dense and orderly perfection like a Beverly Hills lawn. Not so. Some of the sprouts are as downy and transparent as a polar bear's fur, some are the old dark hair cautiously poking above the surface. I could inflict wicked razor burn on someone's soft skin. Her Baldness and I are used to being out and about in the little black cap, and we realize that being bothered by hairlessness depends a great deal on one's emotional and physical state. When I hit bottom, I want hair because hair means energy. Thick short hair means more energy and looks good. This does not answer the question of why Allan Sekula is less startling at an opening in his almost bald pate than I would be in mine, not to mention why—aside from my decision to let the magic marker and emerald green cross hairs from radiation prep show in my cleavage—men at Allan Sekula's stage of alopecia mind their bald pates far less than I mind mine. I feel more inclined now to roll up the front of my cap to show people my returning fuzz, but where I see sprouts they see BALD. No medical person really wants to talk about exactly how hair grows back. In my support group the consensus seems to be that it comes back thicker. Fingernails also get stronger. Realistically we are talking wispy for a few months until I achieve buzz-cut density, though Susun Weed swears that burdock oil and St. John's wort oil are both better than Rogaine, so I will go off to the health food store to have a look.

Various people come up to me to say that I look fabulous. What do you think they're going to say? Kim wonders when I tell her about my evening. WOW! I'd really like to try chemo sometime.

SUNDAY | SEPTEMBER 10, 2000

IN A MESSAGE DATED 9/10/00 JOANAR WRITES: Hey, chemosabe, how are you??

MONDAY | SEPTEMBER 11, 2000

IN A MESSAGE DATED 9/11/00 HEYLORD WRITES: I think that Michael's reaction was right & that she was utterly selfish in laying that information on you, since at some level she must have known the effect it would have. It's as though she's saying, "if I have to die from this thing, I'm going to scare the hell out of as many people as I can along the way."

I think about yoga but don't do it. I have errands but I put them on a list. I have phone calls to make but don't make them. Paperwork to do and I put it off. The writing has no fuel: I am not terrified. Denial? Progress? Pajamas on and house keys in pocket, I am back to 155 pounds, a little below where I started. Kim says that maybe I will have hair back by spring. Early spring, she amends, when I lose it. I worry about Kim's cough.

TUESDAY, | SEPTEMBER 12, 2000

To acknowledge that the whole thing is a crap shoot is no relief. The moment I say out loud to myself that I don't fear death, the fear returns in another guise. And why can't I die? Work not completed? Pleasures yet to be had? Why do I obsess about dying rather than about pain or the loss of bodily control?

IN A MESSAGE DATED
9/12/00 CBLORD@UCI.EDU
WRITES TO UNDISCLOSED
RECIPIENTS:

SUBJECT: HER BALDNESS PREPARES TO GET BURNED

The way it looks now, Radiation Number One will be September 26 and Radiation Number Thirty Three will be November 9, unless I take a day or two off or unless the machines break down in which case Cedars has already apologized in advance for the inconvenience not to mention covered themselves against any possible liability for the cancellation of celebratory festivities. I will go to radiation five days a week. There are people, myself not included, who say that they have been transformed for the better by their cancer and that they wouldn't have missed the journey for the world, but if the trope for this disease is travel, Planet Cancer is an upgrade—valet parking, free oranges and crackers and tea and cappucino in the waiting room, lots of magazines, comfy chairs, people in white coats who lead you from one room to another, and Grant Mudford photographs on the walls. We're talking 24/7 financial counselors, nutritional support, a psychosocial service team, an ambulatory care pharmacy, pain management services, and a library with up to date publications and relaxation tapes. We're talking a 53,000 square foot facility with a brochure about your very own doctor that is mailèd to you before you meet her, and many many expensive machines.

Last week it was my destiny to be inserted into one of them for a CT scan. You lie on a long board on your back. The arm on the side of the breast in question, or rather the breast no longer in question but in deep shit, is placed over your head into a contraption which is basically a piece of particleboard about 20 inches square out of which sprout two metal sticks that support two molded pieces of plastic. One piece of plastic is for the elbow of your bent arm, the other is for the back of your hand. Your arm is thus moved out of harm's way into classic NASA waving-to-the-aliens stance. A technician, in this case named Jim, pushes a button on a schtupper and the whole board slides into the hole in the middle of a large beige plastic donut as high as the ceiling.

The contraption upon which your arm rests might cost twenty bucks. The donut machine costs over a million, minimum, maybe a million and a half, according to my radiation oncologist, Dr. Daphne Palmer.

When she came in to discuss a small discrepancy in my pathology report, I had my legs vertical, bare feet propped on the plastic part of the donut, in order to do a restorative yoga pose while discussing the relative merits of Leicas and Hasselblads with the technician. Multitasking. Well, said Dr. Palmer, looking at my unmanicured Silver Lake lesbian feet on her spotless, million-dollar donut, THAT I haven't seen before. I don't know WHAT the manufacturer would think.

As a beginning, this seemed to me inauspicious. In consequence, I have not yet tried to call Dr. Palmer by her first name. (I outrank her in the University of California system, where she is an associate professor at UCLA, and where we would naturally call each other by our first names. However, the ramifications of transposing professorial collegiality to Cedars are not yet evident to me.) In Dr. Palmer's donut, things spin and whirl and flash while the board goes in and out. Jim used the sort of Sharpie pen you buy at Staples for 59 cents to draw Xs at all four compass points of my RBr. Into the middle of each X he placed small green plastic targets with steel ball bearings in the center. He taped these firmly to my flesh with the medical equivalent of strapping tape and told me everything HAD to stay in place over the weekend until my next radiation planning appointment, four and one half days away.

Come Tuesday morning, me and my cancer that may already have been cured and my itchy pink unwashed skin under the medical equivalent of strapping tape drove over to Cedars to lie under another machine, The Simulator, which cost a lot less than the donut but has the same long board and is designed to mimic the machine that administers radiation. The effect is like being the paper under an old fashioned enlarger. You look up into the enlarger head to a rectangular aperture through which light (and later, radiation) pours. The energy of the beam, that is the depth to which it will penetrate my flesh, is determined by another technician elsewhere in the bowels of the building. This technician I will never meet. This technician will never have a name. His energy level, not MY energy level, is what Jim thinks I should be worrying about, instead of asking a million questions, about, for example, whether the technician I will never meet is a woman.

Jim's work speed is efficient verging on hyper. Another pair of breasts, or perhaps testicles, judging from the population of the waiting room, on the conveyor belt to The Sim. Jim volunteers that when he does this procedure for testicular cancer, he must bring the radiation field along the lymph nodes that run vertically up the belly. As testicular cancer usually falls on one side or the other of the long bar of light Jim creates on the male torso, the template has always looked to him just like a hockey stick. Speaking of which, Jim specialized in product shots when he went to photography trade school, though his heart was really in landscape. As far as the products in his current line of work go, he says, there really isn't much difference between treating floppy middle-aged breasts and young perky ones, or between little breasts and big breasts. Jim's job is to set the radiation rectangle so that it misses as much lung as possible, which means that the real issue is not breast size or breast perk but whether the ribs are bowed or flat. My ribs are bowed, but not as bad as some ribs he has seen.

Even with all this chat, plus a bit more about the pros and cons of point and shoot cameras, it's a long forty five minutes with the back of my neck on hard plastic. When the beam of light comes from below it creates a shadow on the scratched plex screen of the enlarger head that looks like just Ayres Rock in Australia, otherwise known as God's Turd, with an old fashioned rooftop television antenna sticking up out of the summit. Kim, who had at the beginning been photographing The Sim along with the soft flesh of the person inside, is deported to the hall-way, where she watches me through a large window. When she comments to Jim that anyone who walks by can just look in at me and my naked RBr, she is exiled to the waiting room. The reason, Jim says, is that SHE might be exposed to radiation and catch cancer.

Lying in The Sim, I develop a new sympathy for those who sat motion-less for their portraits in daguerreotype days with metal braces to hold their heads and shoulders in place for the long exposures. I salute the ones who made a messy smear across the mirror of memory because they couldn't take it a minute longer no matter how expensive the pho-tograph so they just smiled or laughed or slumped or shook their heads from side to side. Jim tattoos two very small dots on the horizontal axes of my RBr. These dots are permanent. On the matter of tattoos acquired for other, nonfunctional purposes, Jim is emphatically of the school of Adolf Loos: ornament is crime. He takes a few Polaroids of my torso and then sends me off to have a parting chat with Dr. Daphne Palmer, she in her white coat and me in my open-in-the-front Cedars gown.

The pathology report has been resolved. My margins are entirely clear, which is excellent news. I am not to take mega doses of vitamins A, C or E, but I can take green tea and echinacea. My blood count will be done every other week. I should expect fatigue in three weeks or so, though I may experience none at all. I may experience more fatigue at the end of the week than at the beginning. Radiation may cause my skin to thicken and burn, phenomena for which Cedars has its solutions. However, I have comfrey salve on hand and have ordered St. John's wort oil, which Susan Swan the yoga teacher swore got her through the same ordeal with no burn to her fair skin. Or else she could have been lucky: radiation burn, the books say, doesn't depend on the darkness or fairness of skin.

As a backup I have a small brown bottle labeled Huile de Serpent which I bought earlier this year, not knowing to what use I might put it, from a man who sells natural herbs in Roseau. By far his most expensive offering ($15 US for 4 oz.) Huile de Serpent is made by boiling up a kind of boa constrictor called tete de chien. As the tete de chien likes to lie on warm concrete when the sun goes down and the evening turns cool, it is effortlessly harvested from cement roads. There are no radiation facilities on Dominica, so I have no anecdotal evidence as to the efficacy of Huile de Serpent on burns caused by a machine the country cannot afford. Topically administered, however, Huile de Serpent is said to be good for soreness, bruises and skin inflammation. Who knows?

WEDNESDAY | SEPTEMBER 13, 2000

IN A MESSAGE DATED
9/13/00 LORRGRAD WRITES:

To be honest, I cried when I looked at the pictures you sent me. But then I can barely look at myself anymore, and I certainly don't take photos.

ER negative, her2neu expressed. My cancer, indifferent to estrogen, cannot be starved by withhold-ing it. Tamoxifen is not prescribed for ER-negative tumors. My cancer is aggressive. Cause for con-cern. Repeat one thousand times: I do not have a terminal illness diagnosis.

I'm trying, I'm trying, I'm trying, says Kim, meanwhile running late at both ends of the day. I miss her. I miss time with her. I want her to be doing work that means something more than money. We need a beach for our souls. She makes expensive plans for a celebration and I dream of a tacky road trip.

My department chair calls. My medical leave has been extended another quarter.

IN A MESSAGE DATED 9/13/00 CBLORD@UCI.EDU WRITES TO FOCL'SRB:

SUBJECT: NOTES ON SOME THINGS THAT BEGIN WITH B

Beads. When I lived with my family the rule was to put into the neighbor's garbage any object that you never wished to see again. My sister Linda caught the scavenging habit early, and would rummage and grope in trash cans to reappear with old combs, the lenses of eye-glasses, buttons, shoelaces and broken china. These she would hoard until she herself had decided she could bear the separation. As an adult, she is an on-again-off-again dealer in antiques, one of the many women who supplement their income by renting space in an antique mall and selling their findings. She has made it a virtue to have the patience to sort through every bedraggled item in a cardboard box and has in this way accumulated an extensive collection of beads: a handful of ivory here, heavy amber there, garnet, carnelian, amethyst, old silver, tur-quoise, coral and jade. She has an unerring eye. She agreed to bring her collection to Los Angeles with her on her second visit. There were things to repair, things to restring, things to sort. Beading is an indoor activity. Beading is an activity one can do lying in bed. Art therapy, said my mother. It was not an observation intended to encourage. My mother does not believe in psychiatrists.

There were frictions. Linda loves things that involve the killing of ani-mals or substances extracted with difficulty from the earth: old silver, turquoise, ivory. Linda would rather not disperse a collection: pearls should stay with pearls, agate with agate. Linda loves to hold these hard round objects, to roll them in her hand, to stroke them, to wonder at their weight, their cool, hard, unyielding inertia. Linda loves beads more than she loves necklaces, certainly more than she has occasion to wear necklaces. I preferred to proceed by color, shape, and texture, to pick the beads I wanted from whichever little ziplock bag was necessary, and mix them together, no matter whether they were glass or rock crystal or clear plastic. I imagine Linda felt that I wasn't respecting the value of things. I felt that she respected them too much.

So we compromised, though I suspect Linda did more of that than her sister. I lined beads into patterns. Linda strung. Linda allowed rare beads that had spent years in a plastic bag waiting to be separated properly with knots and secured with a safety clasp to rearrange themselves into bracelets on a cheap piece of elastic. Linda permitted the monochromatic mixtures I favored, but she had the veto power over the deployment of any one bead. When it was clear that some combinations disturbed her — coral and plastic, for example — I didn't press. When she felt that some of my combinations had strayed from venturesome to egregious bad taste, she raised her eyebrows only slightly. She held her ground on the matter of two translucent glass beads, old and fogged, on a monochromatic strand of carnelian and agate and amber. I hadn't put them in. She wanted them there. In they went. We looked at each other's wrists and arms and necks and faces in a way we hadn't since we were children and we managed. My sister has beautiful clear pink skin with a light dusting of freckles. She hates her upper arms and has to remind herself, standing in front of the mirror, that they are part of her and that they are to be loved. We didn't talk about what it meant to look at each other as women, and we didn't talk about what it meant to spend days handling hard round objects that can be discussed in gradations of size, but we ended up with more finery than we or anyone we knew could possibly wear.

Beet juice. Last week, as I was walking across the parking lot of the health food store on Hillhurst, drinking my beet juice, a plump woman in her forties hurried to accost me. Excuse me, excuse me, but are you by any chance going through chemo? I had it five years ago, because I had lung cancer bad, and they didn't give me more than a few months. NOW look at me, I'm fine.

Bill Moyers. Her Baldness and I have watched most of the four episodes of *On Our Own Terms,* Moyers' program on the terminally ill, as well as the question and answer bits afterwards. Her Baldness has fash ion issues. She wonders why so few of Moyers' subjects color their hair. Though she is all too aware of the people who look like they have mange and of the women who will die before their short hair grows back in, she estimates that there are more wigs in use than meet the eye. She thinks it is all hopelessly Northern California, and she really wanted to see someone who just couldn't take it and started screaming WHY ME? WHY ME? I'M FUCKING TERRIFIED IT HURTS ALL THE TIME I LOOK LIKE SHIT I DON'T WANT TO DIE MAKE IT ALL THE WAY IT WAS. She looked at a lot of chin wobbling, which comes between tearing up and loud bawling in the sequence of emotional release, and realized that you can't talk while you're crying because the muscles of the jaw and mouth are on a walkout with something related to the sewing machine leg that rock climbers get when they freeze with all their weight on a small fraction of one foot because they cannot figure out where to go next, but if they don't move, they shake themselves off the rock. I completely and totally and porously identify with everyone who is dying, so much so that I have to keep reminding myself that I do not, repeat a thousand times NOT, repeat it again another thousand times, NOT, actually have a terminal diagnosis. I could be in the two-thirds who live, or the one-third who die.

It is, however, unnerving to see people looking pretty much OK, though perhaps a bit pale, and to hear that they died two or three days later. It is just as unsettling to see how strong a habit life is to break. I am using the Moyers program to practice the idea of dying, to prepare myself in case it comes to that sooner than I expect. This is rather like using a treadmill on the steepest incline because you think someday the phone will ring with an invitation to leave for Everest the next week. (Speaking of Everest, Her Baldness hears that 96% of all Americans believe in some kind of God and thinks personally that at least 86% of them are saying so just in case even though, due to the rapidly declining state of our educational system, they never heard of Pascal or of his wager.) Like a sponge or a paper towel, I sop up the idea of dying. It keeps me away from a harder place, which is vividly to imagine living with an extended or possibly a recurrent illness. I am more afraid of dying than I am of chronic pain or physical incapacity, more afraid of fading out, or the final cut, than I am of staying around in the frame as a big motionless drugged object.

Blame. I missed my annual mammogram in 1999. My last mammogram, done in July of 1998, showed nothing abnormal. Every doctor to whom I confess my lapse has been kind. It's not your fault, they say. These things are not detectable and then they are. That's the way it is. There are women who get clear mammograms and then feel their lump a few months later.

Bourgeois, Louise. Hair is simply protection women are wrapped in. Hair is like a caterpillar in a cocoon. But hair is more friendly in that the cocoon eliminates the subject.

Brains. Julia Marie, the massage therapist, keeps a plastic model of a skull in the room she devotes to her cranio sacral work. The room is just off the front porch in the house on a hill in Echo Park that Julia Marie shares with her sister, who should have been dead from cancer four times over, and Grace, who turned a hundred and two just lately. The model is crimson and teal and turquoise and umber. It comes apart, allowing Julia Marie to demonstrate to me, when I ask, why it is she loves the human skull. Julia Marie holds the model tentatively and delicately, as she might a real skull, though she is well aware that it is a mere approximation of the real thing and, in fact, is careful to point out those areas in which the real thing is more beautiful—for instance, the places so thin that they are translucent, the places where the sutures are beveled, and most especially a little place deep inside, right above the spine. For those of you who know and eat your chickens, the place is rather like the concavity of bone on the back where you can pick out that tasty little filet. Julia Marie's favorite place sits above the spine, like an upside down bowl, and cradles the pituitary gland as it hangs from the lobes.

The lobes, Julia Marie says, are not at all firm in the living human being. They do not approach the consistency of jello, or even yogurt. Brains are like soup, she says, and most like kefir. The lobes nestle next to each other like the fruit decoratively arranged in brandy in those Italian jars. Julia Marie works not with the fruit, though she is aware of its softness, but with the brandy, trying to get it to slosh around the fruit in a rocking movement. My brandy isn't rocking. I am exhausted, Julia Marie says. I have been fighting to hold myself together through the chemo, and now there isn't anything left. She doesn't try to bring me back to myself because there is nothing there to be reached.

I, on the other hand, felt for the first time weightless, fearless, buoyant, without a care, floating in the stratosphere of meadows and wildflowers and light.

Breast cancer statistics. 175,000 women were diagnosed with invasive breast cancer in 1999 (1 every 3 minutes). 43,700 people died from breast cancer in 1999 (one every 12 minutes). (*www.breastcanceraction.com*)

Breast, right. It's a cyst, says Ed the surgeon about the lump that has reappeared in the same place as the tumor. Your breasts have softened from the chemo, so the cysts are more obvious. It's normal to have a lump return in the same place that the tumor was removed. I don't want to drain it because of the risk of infection. Also if I drain it you will have a dent. I don't care about the dent, I reply. Just promise me you'll try to make the lump go away when my blood count is back up.

Butler, Judith. In chemotherapy, hair falls from the head because 90% of the hair on the head is in the fast growing, or atagen stage, and so is rapidly affected by the chemicals. Most of the hair in the eyebrows and eyelashes is in the catagen and telogen phases, regression and resting, respectively, and these are unaffected by chemo or radiation except in extremely heavy doses. Hair falls because the protein keratin, which holds the hair shaft to the walls of the follicle, loses its capacity to serve as an anchor. Your hair becomes unglued. It grows back in at the rate of .33 mm per day, or about five inches per year, or much slower than corn. At the moment what I have is hairs. They lack the density to achieve in English the status of a collective singular noun. When I say to people that my hair is growing back I should actually say that some of my hairs are growing back as I am (viz Allan Sekula) still bald. I counted in one section of roughly one square inch six black thick hairs and ten fine white hairs. I can't answer questions about what color my hair will come back because there is as yet, and it may take as long as two years, no collectivity that constitutes a field of color. I am, I suppose, looking at the process of healing, but I am also and simultaneously, in case you were wondering what possible relevance any of this could have to Judith Butler, looking at gender in bud. Gender in bud is not what we usually get to see. Gender in bud is thin paper. Gender in bud is beyond delicate. Gender in bud is flimsy. When you turn up the lights, it's not much of a performance.

FRIDAY | SEPTEMBER 15, 2000

IN A MESSAGE DATED 9/15/00 WHYRAIN WRITES: Are you still coming to NY next week? I'll reserve a restaurant if you want, you name it.

IN A MESSAGE DATED 9/15/00 CROLLO WRITES: your language is really flying. you've hit it so hard, the jello, the amber, the shriek of being sick.

Man on street stops to read parking sign, stops longer to stare at me. A walk on the Santa Monica beach on a weekday afternoon. Have I EVER done this? Empty, peaceful, warm sand, a sandpiper burying its beak and gobbling.

Kevin A. calls. His father did chemo last year. When I say that I'm OK and getting better I can tell that he doesn't believe me.

Group. Facilitator brings up the calendar rebellion. The new BrCa recruit isn't coming back because we were raucous and offensive in our objections to the ceremonial reading of the calendar. The calendar means community and information, she snaps. Community and information will kick start your immune system. This is not a democracy. The calendar is not negotiable. When I fly to New York, she says, I must bring a special bandage to prevent lymphedema in my arm. What's lymphedema? I ask. Swelling. Your whole arm swells and it never comes back to normal. Ed has said nothing of this, or Michael, or Dr. Daphne Palmer. I get angry at the facilitator for dispensing medical advice where she is not qualified. She doesn't have cancer. She never had cancer. What fucking right does she have to occupy so much space?

IN A MESSAGE DATED 9/20/00 CBLORD@UCI.EDU WRITES TO FOCL'SRB:

SUBJECT: TIYA EMET'S TUMOR REDUCING POTION

1 carrot

1 radish

7 calamansi (Philippine/native lemon-lime); lemon will do

Honey or brown sugar

Blend or use juicer. Exclude pulp. Drink before breakfast daily for two weeks; then twice weekly (also before breakfast) for the next two weeks; then once a week (still/as ever before breakfast) thereafter. Sweet fruits (e.g. pineapple, grapes, etc.) may substitute for honey.

(Contributed by Genara Banzon, whose botanist aunt used it successfully for seven months, after which the lump in her throat vanished.)

FRIDAY | SEPTEMBER 22, 2000

New York. The escape between chemo and radiation. Eyebrows went missing when I wasn't paying attention. Lunch with John K. Don't invest too much in your hair coming back, either in quantity or quality. You look pale. He had a friend who never stopped doing work about her breast cancer, so he approves of my desire to get back to the Dominica book.

Exhausted.

SATURDAY | SEPTEMBER 23, 2000

The doctors Kemeny and Nelson assume I will be cured but act like anthropologists with a native informant when I try to explain why I don't want to drink cow's milk. What exactly would be the matter with drinking milk from an animal larger than you are? What makes you think mad cow disease might be transmitted through milk? Why do you think coffee would affect your adrenal glands? The placebo effect is very strong, says Deena politely.

MONDAY | SEPTEMBER 25, 2000

Pate fuzzy to the touch. Hair invisible.

IN A MESSAGE DATED
9/26/00 AVEST WRITES:

Are you feeling better?

A carcinogenic beam aimed at my breast. Thirty-two more. Everyone is back in school. I am the child who remains at home. Last night Kim dreamed people kept staring at me because I had my old hair stuck any which way onto my scalp.

IN A MESSAGE DATED
9/27/00 CBLORD@UCI.EDU
WRITES TO FOCL'SRB:

SUBJECT: HER BALDNESS MEETS BETH AND GETS HIGH ON GENDER

American Airlines, flight 19, JFK to LAX, last Sunday

10:30 a.m., Eastern Standard Time. Her Baldness, upgraded by her gracious and generous and very GIRL (that particular morning) friend from coach to business class and loving her wide window seat with her own blanket and her own pillow says Perrier please while giving the flight attendant her black leather jacket and spilling the Sunday *New York Times*, the real one, the big one, out of a plastic bag, not to mention two thick unillustrated academic books on the history of food, which will of course go unread during the flight, and the latest issue of *Vanity Fair*, which will not.

10:45 a.m. Flight 19 takes off, on time.

11:00 a.m. The flight attendant distributes menus. Pasta involving cream sauce and a lot of cheese, chicken involving a lot of butter, and salad involving a lot of cold beef.

11:15 a.m. The flight attendant, the same flight attendant, a thin white woman in her forties, offers her a choice of drinks. Kim takes club soda with ice and lime. What would you like, sir? the flight attendant inquires of Her Baldness. As Her Baldness has previously encountered gender misidentification, she adopts the pedagogical strategy of nonconfrontation. She manifests enormous indecisiveness about goodies, wavering between mixed nuts and oyster crackers, or both, or neither, or lemon or lime, or ice or not, or flat or sparkling. She settles on club soda, ice, no lime. She is so anxious to give the flight attendant an opportunity to reflect on gender possibilities that she asks for tomato juice in addition to club soda. The flight attendant is amicable, cooperative and patient. Her Baldness congratulates herself on her maturity in using details such as the temperature of a warmed cashew to give the flight attendant an opportunity to reconsider the social construction of gender without provocation or direct criticism. Perhaps, after all, cancer has been a transformative experience for Her Baldness. When the cart rolls off, Her Baldness and the girlfriend agree that the real question is how long it took the flight attendant to change her mind.

11:39 a.m. The flight attendant inquires as to our lunch preferences. As before, she approaches Kim first. Kim votes chicken. The flight attendant turns to Her Baldness. Sir, what will you have this morning? So. Her Baldness has passed from the category of sick female (or possibly, recovering Buddhist nun) into the category of white male. The problem of female baldness has found a solution: disappear female. If bald isn't female, bald is fine. If bald isn't female, bald isn't grotesque. Out there among the clueless heteros, it's easier to see a straight couple than a queer one. The luscious lipstick lesbian, blonde, good haircut, loaded with the signifiers of femme (an identity Kim emphatically rejects) is disappeared into straight woman. The skinny tortured pale butch (an identity to which I, on the other hand, aspire) is disappeared into straight man.

Her Baldness chooses the gourmet salad with slow roasted tomatoes, please hold the chateaubriand and substitute smoked salmon if there is any left after the appetizer course, a long conversation designed to give the flight attendant another opportunity to reflect upon the nuances of gender. Why not try the chicken, CATHERINE? Kim asks. Oh, I forgot, CATHERINE, you're not eating chicken these days.

11:41 a.m. Her Baldness observes, silently, to herself, that in addition to her black cap, she is wearing a wrinkled white man's shirt from the thrift store, black jeans, and Prada shoes that could go either way. She does sport, however, three bead bracelets on the wrist nearest the flight attendant as well as an earring in the ear nearest the flight attendant. Presumably the flight attendant would rather serve a guy who wears bracelets than Her Baldness. Her Baldness decides she is flattered to be called sir.

11.43 a.m. Has Her Baldness unwittingly been sir in New York for the entire week of her cancer vacation? Her Baldness acknowledges that this may well have been the case, with the exception of her friends, who say they find her more fashionable than she used to be, and for Sadie Gund-Hope who said, Catherine, Catherine, stop, Catherine, I want to see your head. Her Baldness felt unbearably shy at this moment. She wanted to run. She was terrified, which made her feel like a freak, as Sadie is only three years old. She showed Sadie the front of her head, but she wasn't brave enough to take off the entire cap. It was hardly one of Her Baldness's finest moments.

12:01 p.m. The flight attendant comes down the aisle with the navy blue polyester tablecloths. Her Baldness is buried in *The New York Times*, reading about how late night talk shows have replaced the news as a source of reliable political commentary. Her Baldness apologizes for the delay in extricating her little plastic food tray from underneath her right armpit. "There's no rush, sir," says the flight attendant. "We've got all the time in the world. The flight is five hours and twenty minutes." Her hair is dyed brown, and she is very thin. Her Baldness tries to make out the flight attendant's name tag but it is obscured by her apron. There are no other same sex couples in business class. Her Baldness wonders who the flight attendant thinks brings home the most bacon in this straight couple—the femme who is used to ordering club soda and lime or the guy in bracelets.

12:03 p.m. Reality check. Ever since Her Baldness handed over her leather jacket on Flight 19, she has been a sir. But isn't Her Baldness a VERY smooth shaven guy? Or does the flight attendant think she's a depilatory minded fag? Or an F2M?

12:12 p.m. The flight attendant rolls the cart to the front of the cabin. Time for wine and the tossed green salad with smoked salmon. The flight attendant puts on her glasses so that she can read the labels.

12:14 p.m. Kim observes that flight attendants live in a bubble. They are totally out of touch with the sort of popular culture of which bald people in black knit caps are an example.

12:35 p.m. Kim's chicken arrives, along with Her Baldness's two slow roasted tomatoes, four pieces of asparagus, and half a piece of smoked salmon, the exact provenance of which Her Baldness, who still has an iffy sort of immune system, prefers not to consider. The flight attendant, who is no longer wearing her glasses, turns to Kim first. Ma'am, would you like anything else? Excuse me, please, says Her Baldness, could I possibly have a bit more club soda? Her Baldness thinks she's getting positively girlish about the way she strings words into sentences and, in her head, tries to rehearse a more manly way to get the club soda off the cart. More club soda please. That would have sufficed. Her Baldness puts on her own glasses. BETH. That's what the name tag says. Her Baldness takes hummus and crackers out of her backpack.

12:38 p.m. Of course, I am not wearing lipstick today.

12:39 p.m. I have worn lipstick perhaps twice in the last five years.

12:41 p.m. Her Baldness wonders whether BETH's patience with her many requests is in fact an effect of being a guy. Perhaps Her Baldness is sufficiently manly, in her quiet and understated way, to obviate the need for anyone actually to utter the word sir. Her Baldness conceives of this as the deployment of male privilege. She rather likes feeling the ripple effect, which she visualizes as the way the muscles of the abdomen roll when those who have them use them.

12:46 p.m. Today's movie is *Here on Earth*. Gorgeous working-class babe falls while running. There's something I've been meaning to tell you, she confesses to rich boyfriend. Oops. Cancer.

12:52 p.m. While she was in New York, Her Baldness checked out Nancy Burson's "Race Machine" at Exit Art. You sit in a little booth. You line the corners of your eyes up against two cross hairs. You are scanned. Afterwards you get a choice of five menu items: White, Black, Asian, Hispanic, and Indian. Nancy Burson is not particularly critical of the social construction of race or gender. Nancy Burson has worked for the FBI to help them figure out how what certain of their Most Wanted would look like if they changed sex. When Her Baldness pushes White she looks unrecognizably femme. When she pushes Black she looks recognizably male. She likes the idea that the Race Machine, by showing white as something foreign to white people, might get them to denaturalize their racial category. Her Baldness realizes that BETH is unaware she lives in a Gender Machine.

1:06 p.m. BETH removes the trays. She asks whether she should leave the navy blue polyester tablecloths for dessert. Yes, says Kim and YES, says Her Baldness, who immediately regrets her enthusiasm. Her craving for sugar might dissolve the shiny patina of male privilege. Her Baldness wants those abs. She may have blown her cover. Or perhaps Her Baldness's interest in whether BETH reads her as male or female is in itself a feminizing sort of hormone.

1:08 p.m. It is true that Her Baldness is in business class and that she is wearing a black hooded sweatshirt on top of the big man's shirt. She doesn't look like a suit. However it is Sunday and though everyone is white, no one is wearing a suit. Her Baldness wonders whether the bulk of the Sunday New York Times obscured Beth's view of the breast signifier from the outset.

1:11 p.m. BETH needs glasses to see the labels on the wine.

1:21 p.m. BETH comes by to offer macadamia nut ice cream and pie of some sort, as well as coffee, tea and after dinner drinks. Her Baldness refuses everything, but Her Baldness is too fucking accommodating. No, thank you very much, instead of no thanks. The girlfriend is an emphatic ma'am. Her Baldness doesn't rate a sir. Her Baldness is a gender nothing.

1:23 p.m. On the David Letterman show, a cross between a golden retriever and a dalmatian catches balls in a baseball glove.

1:31 p.m. Her Baldness heads for the bathroom, minus her black sweatshirt. She does a few yoga stretches and sticks her chest out. Her Baldness has two fair-sized knockers. BETH is very helpful in explaining the exact location of the bathroom.

2:15 p.m. BETH comes by again. Would you like anything more to drink, sir? Perhaps Her Baldness is an academic male, the vegan sort, of minor fame. Her Baldness asks for club soda. You must have drunk a whole bottle of club soda already, CATHERINE, says Kim, who is completely exasperated with BETH and therefore has a fit of protectiveness. She has been trying to shield Her Baldness from gender insult for almost four hours. I don't want you to correct her, says Her Baldness when BETH goes off. I WANT to be sir for five hours and twenty minutes. I'd rather be a bald white guy with bracelets than a sick white woman.

2:17 p.m. What is it that BETH can't spell. L.E.S.B.I.A.N. or C.H.E.M.O.?

THURSDAY | SEPTEMBER 28, 2000

IN A MESSAGE DATED
9/28/00 WHYRAIN WRITES: BETH is totally unfamiliar with both L.E.S.B.I.A.N and C.H.E.M.O. As your femmie partner said, she lives in a bubble of misrecognition. Interesting that you were able to get some satisfaction out of passing. I never do, maybe because I've never allowed myself to let the instrument of such passing get away with it for very long. I always disabuse the erring flight attendant (who, by the way, is usually female; if it's a male, and he is in doubt, he will omit any gendered address). Something puritan in me feels guilty in the face of deception. Also, telling them before they "find me out" on their own is important to my sense of retaining the upper hand.

IN A MESSAGE DATED 9/28/00 JMK WRITES: Forget Her Hirsuteness. Her Baldness is morphing into His Baldness.

Exhaustion by 1:30 p.m. I am only on my third radiation. This cannot be.

FRIDAY | SEPTEMBER 29, 2000

IN A MESSAGE DATED 9/29/00 VOLT WRITES: ca m'a bien fait rigolé, sir.

IN A MESSAGE DATED 9/29/00 SEC WRITES: The gay men are all shaving their heads to mystify their baldness/aging effects, so you were probably passing as a gay man, who was trying to pass as a young man. Just think, as you try to look more and more indecisive and "girlish"—BUTCH BOTTOM!

SATURDAY | SEPTEMBER 30, 2000

Borders? Nuances? What's the difference between bald and short hair, between sick and Marine, between Marine and gym teacher, between gym teacher and dyke?

Did the Landa steps today, all 236, the first time in four months.

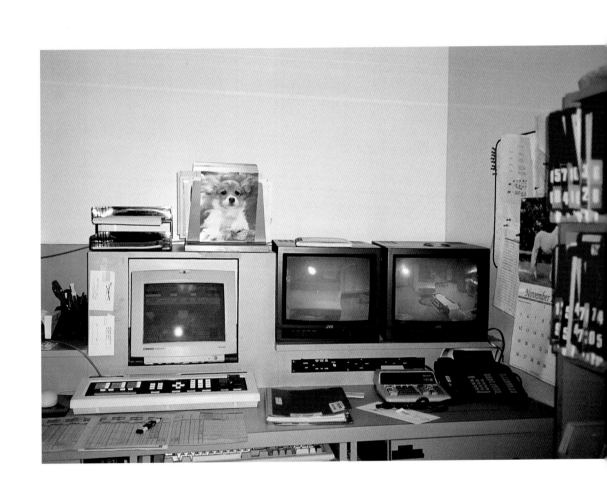

OCTOBER | 2000

Hollywood farmer's market. Corn and peppers and eggplant and squash and French tulips and swordfish and hummus and cristophine and basil and thyme and arugula. Such bounty. Dee Dee the heirloom tomato pioneer asks where I have been. I come out. It turns out her mother died of breast cancer a few years ago. She forgets to give me back the quarter she always gives me for my artist's IRA.

MONDAY | OCTOBER 2, 2000

IN A MESSAGE DATED
10/2/00 SUSANF WRITES:

what's your schedule like on tuesday or wednesday evenings? i have this vagina dentata melon for you from the louvre.

IN A MESSAGE DATED
10/2/00 LORRGRAD WRITES:

I loved your latest missive. It reminded me of the kind of ambiguity I've lived with all my life (less since I stopped straightening my hair). I'm glad you have somebody who wants to protect you from it.

TUESDAY | OCTOBER 3, 2000

IN A MESSAGE DATED
10/3/00 CBLORD@UCI.EDU
WRITES TO UNDISCLOSED
RECIPIENTS:

SUBJECT: HER BALDNESS BEGINS A SLOW BURN

It's not bad so far at Planet Cancer, six radiations down and twenty-seven to go, blood count just fine, thank you (4100 WBC and hemoglobin 14.2, not to mention 217 on the platelets), so fine that I can get a flu shot and go to the dentist. In fact, at the moment it's hard to think of radiation as anything more difficult than the chore of driving halfway across Los Angeles at rush hour. The seniority system rules at Planet Cancer. I began with 7:30 a.m., moved to 9:15 a.m. in a few days, when a guy with prostate phased out, and will nail the 11:45 a.m. slot by the end of this week, unless the woman who now occupies it turns out to need a boost. I can then circle until the 3.30 p.m. clears for landing, giving me a full day to work before I go to Cedars. Nothing visible is happening to my breast that would let me know it is being irradiated. Except for a few microscopic tattoos and the fact that I lie on a long tray powered by a hydraulic lift under a large contraption that points at my breast, first from the medial side and then from the lateral, and buzzes like mad for about thirty seconds on each side, the entire medical intervention is abstract.

Nothing stings, nothing hurts. I feel stronger and stronger every day. Being strong enough to drive to Planet Cancer and back, by myself, makes me deliriously happy. The weed killer is leaving my system and so far the fatigue I am supposed to feel from radiation is caused from the drive to the machine, which takes longer than aligning the machine to the particulars of my breast, which in turn takes longer than the radiation itself. Everyone associated with the machine is nice. Henry at the check in counter, Darrin the friendly technician, Luisa who sticks me for blood, and Martha the chief nurse, who is comforting in the way that women in their sixties who have seen it all are comforting. You'll recover, you're young and strong. Make sure to rub this cream in three times a day.

There is the predictable skin hierarchy: Henry, the receptionist, is a dark brown African American, Martha and Dr. Daphne Palmer, the highest paid, are very white Caucasian. In between Henry and Daphne lie the technicians—Latino and Filipino. (Two machines are in operation at all times, from 6:30 a.m. until 7 p.m., says Darrin, meaning roughly 100 patients per day, and that is not, says he, as many as Kaiser Permanente, which treats about 250 patients a day.)

The biggest trouble I have with radiation, so far, is the idea of doing the same thing five days a week at more or less the same time. Every night I worry that I'll just forget to go the next day. Perhaps this fear is typical of novitiate analysands, and in that case the idea of transference might apply. Though it is a relief and oddly comforting, however, to have SOMETHING, even if only a machine, pay attention to my breast, what the machine is doing is as yet invisible and I can't really manage to smear it with the fertile muck of old infantile attachments to authority. When I asked Dr. Palmer how much of a dose I was getting each day, she said a perfectly average 180 RADS, or radiation absorbed density. How many RADS in a mammogram? I asked. She thought maybe one. That makes each morning's zap the equivalent of 180 mammograms, for a total, over 33 treatments, of 5,940 mammograms. You will get a burn, said Dr. Palmer. If you had larger breasts you would get a worse burn, as we would need more radiation to get through the breast tissue. The burn will have absolutely clean edges. She drew the shape of the rectangle that will turn pink on the polaroid mug shots of my breast that Jim the ex-photographer had stapled to my file.

Radiation works, Dr. Palmer says, by reacting with the water in your body to form free radicals, which damage the DNA in your cells in all areas that the radiation touches. The DNA in your skin and glands recovers quickly, usually in the 24 hours between the radiation treatments. But cancer cells are permanently damaged. To say it differently, normal cells have a repair mechanism, and cancer cells do not, so they cannot regenerate after they have been attacked by radiation. Conceptually, then, radiation is as crude an assault on the body as chemo, which kills all the good fast growing cells, like hair follicles and white blood cells and the linings of the mucous membranes, in order to kill the bad fast growing cells, like cancer.

Chemo is like using a cannon to shoot a mouse, said Dr. Peggy Kemeny as we were walking down Twelfth Street in New York the week before last. It's not satisfactory and we will come up with something better soon. BUT, she hastened to add, the cannon kills the mouse.

These are the things one considers, lying five feet up in the air on the radiation bed while the machine moves in an arc and then buzzes to show it is doing its stuff. Whatever I am or am not projecting onto the machine, it is transferring onto me something strong enough to fog the film in my camera and permanently burn my skin. Darrin, who is 24 years old and knows me as Miss Lord rather than Her Baldness, lets me photograph the machine when I am under it, and then moves the camera safely out of the way before he goes into the other room to turn on the radiation. Something strong enough to fog my film when I try to look straight into its eye but that I nevertheless cannot see sounds like a perfect description of the nuclear family, come to think of it, so perhaps there's more material here than I am recognizing.

Hairwise, the sides are looking thin but good, coming up white and lying down flat. The top is thinner, and stands straight up. The location of the line between bald and extremely short hair, particularly when much of that hair is white and therefore barely visible against white skin, eludes me. The skin on my scalp still feels screamingly exposed and blindingly white: white therefore sick therefore white. As I don't like the meaning of either, "sick" or "white," especially when they rotate in a vicious circle, I am trying to get a little tan, hoping it will color me less sick and thus less white, but I think my efforts will soon be rendered moot by hair. On the other hand, as has been gently pointed out to me, invasive treatments for breast cancer mean facing the matter of aging. The hair that is covering the white skin I don't much like is white.

This morning in the parking lot of Planet Cancer I ran into a woman who had been in the radiation waiting room exactly a week ago. I could make out just the shape of a hairline, rather than anything that added up to hair. Now Alison has a distinguished-looking crew cut that would do any self-respecting dyke proud, though she isn't, I am sure, a dyke. She has a thick fuzzy dense head of gray and black, and EYEBROWS. "Look at you," she said, inspecting my fuzz. "Last week you were bald! It happens REALLY quickly." Alison's last chemo was ten days before mine, so Her Baldness is thinking that in a couple of weeks she'll be dealing with a name change.

Her Baldness went to an art world event last night, Komar and Melamid at LA County Museum of Art. Awful but packed. (The trouble is that now, when Alex Melamid pretends to be reading from a script that says, "I am a genius," he believes it.) Her Baldness was looked through, that is to say, went entirely unrecognized, by five people she knows professionally and has had meals with—a curator, a writer, an artist, a professor at another UC campus and a writer. Not even a turn of the head. Having lately had a bit of practice with this sort of thing, Her Baldness took a certain pleasure in her disappearance. She didn't flail her arms and try to surface. She sank with pleasure.

I've been very far away and I'm not ready to return.

I drive hatless to Planet Cancer and back, though I keep my hat next to me on the seat, in case.

Of what?

Salmon on fire in the barbecue. Broccoli too hard to wash. I am losing my mind with depression. Hair coming back white. No stubble on top, just at back. Berate myself about what I haven't done in my life. Stare. Trouble weeding.

Group: On the way out I catch myself in the bathroom mirror and drive back home weeping. I hate being bald. I hate being a freak. I hate being sick. Kim is not home from dinner and I sit on the sofa and bawl. When she gets back I manage to ask about taking the whole week at Thanksgiving.

Kim is stretched thin. Kim can't fix this. Shrink starts to cry. You're not in trouble, she says. You're just having a hard time.

I feel like a failure because I caught cancer. Don't put yourself down, says shrink. Be compassionate. Don't go there.

IN A MESSAGE DATED 10/6/00 CBLORD@UCI.EDU WRITES TO UNDISCLOSED RECIPIENTS:

SUBJECT: HER BALDNESS WAKES UP AND SMELLS THE ROSES

Her Baldness has taken the position, this week, the week that Milosevic was ousted and for once the front page of the newspaper was cause to rejoice, that hair is a state of mind, a performance, a sign of agency, the code and the instrument of pleasure. A dildo. And she has been wanting to take out that dildo for a while, or at least to remember where in the closet she shelved it. She can't remember what it would be like to use one or to feel able to be vulnerable to one, or to a hand, or to a tongue, but that's another story. She has been going unhatted since Tuesday last on her various expeditions, namely to Planet Cancer and to the supermarket and to the health food store and on walks about the neighborhood and to the movies, not to mention to her support group. Group applauded when she walked in on Thursday night, which is not the reaction HB gets at the supermarket, where she is ignored, or at

Planet Cancer, where the reaction to her unhatted pate is affectionate and congratulatory but less audible. In most lights the pate doesn't shine anymore, though there remains a lot of white skin showing through the silver hair. Her Baldness has a hair line, if not exactly hair, form if not content. Form can be a lot more than content. Form can be everything. Form is content. Her Baldness is down with that.

Are you trying to prove something by going out without your hat? asked Kim. Yes. You don't have to.

Here are other commonly asked questions. Is Her Baldness a means of making light of something very serious? Yes. Also no. Her Baldness knows this is serious, believe me. Also her. Everything will be OK, right? You are getting better. Maybe. Her Baldness can be pretty miserable sometimes: scared, needy, weepy, etc. When will Her Baldness depart from this world? Not necessarily when Catherine grows back her hair. There are many forms of cohabitation. There have been issues of negative transference with the shrink and I am thinking that Her Baldness and I might be a better match.

At Planet Cancer a sign has gone up by the elevator announcing OC-TOBER IS BREAST CANCER AWARENESS MONTH, a splendid example of preaching to the converted. Will the other kinds of cancer get their turn? August and September haven't been colonized by other body parts but maybe November will turn out to be, say, STOMACH CANCER AWARENESS MONTH and get its own ribbon. Puce? Aubergine? In the waiting room at radiation, one floor down, everyone wears hospital gowns with a small blue floral pattern. The gowns are quite short and designed to tie in the back. We tie them in the front. Lots of flesh shows, mainly ten or twenty years older than mine. On women, things above the waist flop out. On the men things below the waist hang out. For those of you who don't know, Her Baldness is here to testify that women are not afflicted with their own special kind of fat. MEN HAVE CELLULITE. Also thigh dimples. Also sag. What seems remarkable in this room of seasoned flesh are the young—a small dark girl child asleep on a gurney, her mother beautiful beside her—and those new to the game, tense, fearful, anxious, unto themselves, sitting up straight, afraid to look into the eyes of those who have grown accustomed to their cancer, all the ties of their hospital gowns in neat bows, there at 10 a.m. because that's when the new ones get their CT scans and their port films. The old timers give the new ones room, noticing but not talking, hinting at the opportunity for a smile rather than offering an actual smile, because that would call for a response. It's respect for the memory of one's own raw fear.

In my support group the recently diagnosed are ingested by a more structured process. The newest person is Tom, a film industry something in his seventies whose perfectly put together wife attends the family and friends group that meets next door. Tom is the only man in the group, and we welcome him by going around the room and giving the *Reader's Digest* version of our pathologies. It goes like this, using myself as the example. I was diagnosed with stage IIA breast cancer at the end of May. I had a 1.5 cm tumor and one positive node. I had a lumpectomy and a lymph node dissection. I had chemo for three months and now I am doing a seven-week course of radiation. Everyone takes her turn, and then the newcomer gets all the time she needs to spill her guts.

Tom has inoperable pancreatic cancer. He has lost thirty pounds. He used to be a fine fellow, fit and strapping. I don't much like Tom, though I feel ashamed that I don't because things do not look good for Tom. Tom refers to women as girls. He tries to prevent us from engaging in what he calls bickering by raising his voice. His wife cooks for him, as she always has. He doesn't have a clue that there might be anything wrong with this. His legs are like twigs and he complains because his stomach sticks out to a point because of the scars and he has to buy his pants extra large now and wear suspenders to keep them up. He is a mess from his chest to his pubic hair and he is convinced he is repulsive to his wife. He feels excluded from group unless he is talking and all the women are paying attention to him. I feel, ludicrously and self-righteously and anachronistically and arrogantly, that the women are participating in their own oppression. Down with the patriarchy, I want to scream. Très seventies. Bad for the immune system.

At the last group Tom asked me how many chemos I had had. Four, I replied. Is that ALL? he exclaimed. I get one every week and it doesn't bother me at all. The other women, Doris and Leslie and Naomi, took him on. Your chemo is different, they said to Tom. The chemo we had for breast cancer takes it out of you. It takes three weeks to get you to the point where they can give it to you again without endangering your life. IT WIPES YOU OUT COMPLETELY. It brings you to the bottom and then you come back up slowly and it wipes you out again. The women didn't attack and they didn't get angry. They were polite and they took care of me without saying that they were doing so and without suggesting to Tom that he apologize, though he did so later, and I accepted his apology. I didn't know, he said. Mine isn't like that. I have decided not to die, he announced at the end of group, because I have learned from you valiant ladies. Women will do fine, muttered the facilitator. Tom didn't hear her.

Doris the customs officer is particularly good at handling Tom. Her specialty is drug busts, big ones, and she is trained to spot the cracks in a façade, the small tremors of doubt, the trickle of dust that indicates the beginning of the avalanche. Take eye movements, for example. Looking up to the right is more significant than looking up to the left, because it means that the suspect is looking to the creative side of the brain to find a lie. People who put their hands in front of their faces are trying to push a lie back in. Once in group I tried to explain away my red ears by pleading chemo-induced menopause. No way, said Doris. The rest of your face isn't red. If we were at the airport, I would have pulled you off line. Doris is a pro. No matter how frothy the conversational distractions, Doris remembers the key phrase, word for word, and circles back. She no longer carries a gun on the job because neuropathy, the tingling and numbness in the extremities that can be a side effect of certain kinds of chemo, has affected her ability to feel the trigger.

I know I look fine, she throws out, and people always say to me I look fine, but I am still sick. Ovarian cancer is a death sentence. I have the bones of a 65 year old woman and I am only 46. My hips hurt when I stand up. Cancer took 20 years away from me. Here is where they put a port into my arm and here is where they cut away the veins to get the IV in and here is where the surgical tape that I turned out to be allergic to ripped all the skin off my arm. I have a scar that runs the length of my stomach and I can't lose the thirty pounds I gained during chemo and I can't imagine being attractive to any man and no I am not having sex. My priority is life-sustaining activities. Sex is not a life-sustaining activity.

Customs is a family, she remarks a few minutes later, loudly. She got nine months off because people she didn't know who worked in customs all over the world transferred their leave time to her. Now Doris is wondering why she didn't take disability retirement when it would have been easy for her. She is an overachiever and except that she attaches male pronouns when referring, vaguely, to her past sex partners I frankly do not see how this woman can be straight. She lent me a cancer book so that I could look at the drawings—breasts and flaps and labia and little clits. Better than regular porn, she said. Perhaps that's the customs officer in her. Perhaps she would bust the book if it tried to come across the border. Anyway, everybody seems to be in the land of virtual sex except Naomi who has more scars than anyone because she has Crohn's disease in addition to breast cancer and who associates her scars with the friends who loved her through each operation.

People phrase their facts differently. My doctor, said Tom, gave me three or four months. Suzie prefers "if I die." Her doctor told her she will, though this is a prognosis she revealed to the group just a few weeks ago. Her chemo has been stopped because her tumor is not shrinking. She is stick thin and giving away her clothes. She has married her boyfriend of seventeen years and is making financial arrangements so that she no longer has to think about money. She wants to protect her boyfriend because he isn't very good about money and he doesn't want to talk about death with her which makes her so lonely that she weeps in group. I have stroked her back at these times and she patted the incipient fuzz on my head last week when I cried in fear and desperation and depression that it wasn't over yet and that I had five more weeks of radiation and that even though I felt better I couldn't trust it because I felt just fine before the whole ordeal, excuse me journey, began, so the lesson I have learned is never to trust my body again.

Kim dreamed this week that I was sitting on the sofa with beautiful long red hair, shoulder length red hair. We were both happy. When she put me under the light to admire my hair, it was gone. She woke up crying because she couldn't fix it. In my dreams I have hair, long hair, brown hair, wavy hair, my former hair. As I wake into the memory of cancer, I go bald. In the search to find a disease against which I could vaccinate myself, I got a flu shot this week and pushed Kim to get one too so that I could vaccinate myself against her future as well. It knocked me over for a few days, physically and emotionally, and as a result I tumbled into despair. The thing is, I said to a friend who asked me why I sounded so sad, the thing is that I still have cancer.

Get a wig or cover the mirrors, said the shrink. Do not stay where you are. You cannot afford it. Tough love. Kim plans little trips and I plan big fantasy trips but no matter how far we plan to go in celebration of it being over no plane flies there. The best mode of transportation is more like walking and it will take time to go the distance back to where other people live. Illness is a place, said Flannery O'Connor, who knew. Kim is with me in that place. It's getting on to four and a half months.

So when the going gets tough, the tough read catalogues. Bloomingdale's, for instance, Winter 2000. KAREN NEUBURGER WAKE UP AND SMELL THE ROSES BREAST CANCER AWARE-NESS PAJAMAS. *An important message for an important cause.* Button front top with polo collar; 2 patch pockets. Pull-on, elastic waist pant. Double brushed for softness inside and out. Pink. Cotton/polyester. Imported. Misses S,M,L,XL. $64.00 White with pink floral pattern and pink breast cancer ribbon.

SUNDAY | OCTOBER 8, 2000

Fifteen-minute naps have stretched to a few hours.

MONDAY | OCTOBER 9, 2000

IN A MESSAGE DATED 10/9/00 CBLORD@UCI.EDU WRITES TO UNDISCLOSED RECIPIENTS:

SUBJECT: RECENT SELECTED ACCESSIONS (MORE), COLLECTION OF HER BALDNESS

Her Baldness is immensely grateful, in separate and particular ways, for the following, though she has been slow in getting around to saying so.

Michael Downing, *Breakfast With Scot*

Wooden kaleidoscope

Small woven covered basket and four soft linen pillowcases

Eye mask that can be frozen and Cambridge Census 2000 T-shirt

Several checks for $75 to help with Julia Marie

One pair Prada shoes, one pony-skin bag from Barney's and two nights at Shutters

One certificate for a hair color appointment

One polychrome wooden figure from Hanoi

One white T-shirt with INVERT, in pink, stenciled upon a yellow oval in the center of the chest

Large yellow teapot and tin of green tea

One Thai massage

One round red squishy object stamped with the word PROCRIT

One pin in the shape of a pink ribbon

One white T-shirt with femme-ish sheep jumping over a fence above the word CAUTION.

TUESDAY | OCTOBER 10, 2000

Nancy calls, wanting to talk about her house on stilts in a marsh. Do you feel awful? No. Her mother died of cancer but I do not remember what kind. Nancy made drawings.

Lisa calls. I cannot convince her that I am not actually dying. Am I too sick? Not sick enough?

I am needy. Kim enables. For the strength of the relationship, she needs to set limits. Wispies about an inch long in unpredictable places.

IN A MESSAGE DATED
10/11/00 CBLORD@UCI.EDU
WRITES TO UNDISCLOSED
RECIPIENTS (UNSENT):

SUBJECT: COLLECTION OF HER BALDNESS, DEPARTMENT OF REMARKS THAT MIGHT BE RECONSIDERED

I hope your next chemotherapy is as uneventful as the last.

You're not going to die.

Those odds sound pretty good.

I can see you're going to milk this for all it's worth.

Try not to be morbid.

You will get better.

This is the worst summer of my entire life. I don't think I can take anymore.

You are better.

I want to come over and talk about me.

You look better.

I was so pissed I could have pulled my hair out.

I liked you with short hair but it makes you look more like a lesbian.

I thought that lesbians didn't mind being bald.

I shaved my head in India and I loved it.

THURSDAY | OCTOBER 12, 2000

The burn is worst at the end of the week. This is Thursday and I have the burn I would get lying in the midday sun for fifteen minutes after a long winter.

FRIDAY | OCTOBER 13, 2000

IN A MESSAGE DATED
10/13/00 MRLADY WRITES:

I still attempt to control things by placing good and bad thoughts into the atmosphere according to my whims and wishes. And my wish is for you to be healthy and safe - so my thoughts are with you. Please don't hesitate if there is anything I could possibly do for you.

Hair long enough to need light pruning, hats something I need only for warmth.

Why doesn't chemo obviate the need for radiation, I ask Dr. Palmer. No one knows. But survival rates are about 15–20% more with radiation. The statistics doctors throw at me never add up to a hundred.

SUNDAY | OCTOBER 15, 2000

Marta calls to express her sympathy. You've done pretty well for yourself, she says. A girlfriend with a BMW and an apartment in New York.

Would she like to trade places?

MONDAY | OCTOBER 16, 2000

IN A MESSAGE DATED
10/16/00 SHARHA WRITES:

sulfur you need foods with sulfur in them to get rid of the effects of radiation. brussels sprouts, garlic, cabbage, horsetail supplements.

im still looking for a crap job. ive been interviewed for crap now 4 times. i put on my monkey suit 4 times. i quit one on friday night as my feet were bleeding and they were making us carry loads over 40 lbs. i'm too old . . . my fucking back is out. i was getting paid 9.75 an hour no tips so i thought i'd rather clean toilets in private homes for 10. its hard as i'm too old to waitress in this so called town. its a long boring story but true, and i'm even lying and saying im 34. i thought 34 was still a reasonable age/image but nope. so im broke, spent my money on stupid practical (but quite lovely) waiter shoes that kill, cruel shoes, mens 8's but my feet are deformed . . . from waitressing . .

am i cheering you up????????

Julia Marie doesn't think I have hair.

Last week there was a stain on the couch. Piss. Chloe the cat was the immediate suspect. Perhaps, since she has cancer, too, this was a sign of her final decline. On the other hand, Chloe was sleeping a beatific and untroubled sleep in her basket and one of my exes, who had decided to visit after this diagnosis, had been sitting in that exact spot before she left. My ex is getting on to seventy. Perhaps it was the final judgment of her judgmental visit, in which she took issue with the size of my car (an SUV), my previous haircut (it looks like an art historian), my current haircut (it looks like you had cancer), and the color of my clothes (black). She returned a catalogue of mine for a show called Gender, *fucked. Not my cup of tea, she said. Perhaps, said Kim's mother, whose unconscious dislikes me, it was Catherine who peed on the couch. What about all those drugs she's been taking?*

TUESDAY | OCTOBER 17, 2000

IN A MESSAGE DATED
10/17/00 CBLORD@UCI.EDU
WRITES TO VOLT:

my mood swings suck. les vacances seem very far away. we are getting to paris the 21st of december. will you be around? we invite you to a fabulous dinner.

To Irvine for the Beall Center opening.

IN A MESSAGE DATED
10/17/00 CBLORD@UCI.EDU
WRITES TO UNDISCLOSED
RECIPIENTS:

SUBJECT: NOTES ON SOME THINGS BEGINNING WITH S
Sarah. Rob, who works down the hill at Red Lily, a plumbing establishment this house knows all too well, arrived a few weeks ago to deduce the location of the water leak that had sent our bills skyrocketing, found it in the worst possible and therefore most expensive place, and called me out of my studio to talk about it, which brought us onto the subject of the life expectancy of pipes. Rob says that pipes made before World War II last longer than pipes do now because the detonation of approximately 1,000 nuclear weapons since World War II has affected the atomic structure of metals. There's a lot of radiation in the air and pipes don't last as long as they used to. All that radiation isn't so good for people either, he says. He's tall and thin and red haired and he tells Chloe the cat she is beautiful. Looks like you're going through chemo, he says to me. Finished, say I, and we high five each other.

This brings us to Rob's theory of cancer, which he illustrates with the leaves and seed pods of the Chinese elm under which we are sitting. The tiny yellow leaves are radiation and the little green seed pods are the cells. There are a lot of yellow leaves falling and they get between the green seed pods. Some of the green seed pods are OK but some of them decide they've had it, they're just going to get smothered before they can reproduce, which is what they were put on earth to do, so they jump ship, they just get together and LEAVE the part of the body that they ought to be a part of and they go off and reproduce all by themselves. Rats and the sinking ship? I ask. Yes, says Rob. And it happens first in the reproductive organs, with testicular cancer and prostate and ovarian. He leaves the word breast out of his inventory of reproductive tissues. Finally I realize he can't say breast in front of me, so I say it, BREAST, but even then or perhaps especially then Rob can just barely manage. He has a faint Canadian accent. The reproductive organs are the places that are most convinced of the need to get on with it, to preserve their genetic code. It's their mission. When something threatens them, they react fast. We agree on copper pipe for $840. How come you've thought about this so much? I ask. It was Sarah and Jordan, he says. They were my aunts and they died way before their time. Sarah was the hardest. She gave it up at forty-eight, and she had been fighting it since her twenties, and she never really had the chance to live her life. I had to read up about cancer, he explains. When I look at him in the midst of his arrangement of green seed pods and yellow leaves, his eyes are tearing up. I won't charge you for this discussion, he promises when we say goodbye.

Scratching. Don't, say the women in my support group. Put signs up everywhere in your house. DO NOT GIVE IN. When your skin burns it itches and if it itches you want to scratch but if you scratch and your skin breaks they won't give you any more until it heals and then you will just have to wait longer for it to be over. So far, getting on to half-way through, I show the very beginning of two of the corners of the rectangle made by the radiation beam and these are visible only if I hold my arm exactly in the position, basically the hello-to-visitors-from-another-planet position, in which I lie to receive the beam.

Shadow. Pubic hair, when it returns, begins as fuzz on the outer labia and rises slowly to fill the triangle.

Shame. Her Baldness didn't really know she spent her summer as an apprentice drag queen, or king, but she did. Her Baldness was, she sees now that she is moving to the status of a has-been, all about getting over shame, only she wasn't as informed about it as a drag queen, or king. It is, however, hard to be bald and proud when you feel like shit. Also, the thing about cancer, in case I haven't made this perfectly clear, is the stigma that attaches to it. To be sick with cancer is somehow to have failed—at managing stress, at inheriting the right genes, at strengthening the immune system. To have cancer is often to catch people wondering how soon you will die. It is easier to perform bald (i.e., a voluntary shave) than to be bald, easier in this case to have than to be. Perhaps this is what M2Fs feel about drag queens. Conversely, to have hair is entirely a leap of faith. People who don't see me much say my hair is growing back nicely. I say it has grown back.

Shrink. When I dropped my sunglasses behind the couch in her office, I discovered where my shrink keeps her shit: toys, old packages, pictures frames, bubble wrap.

Sir. I used to think that to be called Sir was either a sign of hostility to me as a lesbian, or an indication that a clueless member of the heterosexual public was groping with the fact that something about me was different but couldn't quite manage to retrieve the word "lesbian" from his or her database. The latter I often took as a compliment. The other day, at the intersection of Virgil and Temple, driving Kim's BMW, the African-American man in his fifties standing on the median line to whom I gave a couple of dollars said thank you, sir. I realized that functionally I was, as a white person with very short hair in a very expensive car, definitely a sir. I had passed from white lesbian with cancer to white man with BMW. Given my choices, I didn't mind being a man.

Sleep. If the sleep I now sleep is what is meant by radiation fatigue, it is a glorious thing. Chemo sleep was fitful, thin, patchy. It was the body's escape from pain, a collapse punctuated by waking into fear. These days, radiation days, I find myself waking up from a two-hour nap after I have stretched out for a moment to read a book. I sleep the sleep of a child. I go down trusting that I will wake, and that I will feel stronger when I do. I wake smiling, trying to put a name to an unfamiliar state which I am coming to recognize as simply feeling rested. Except for the pink skin, which now, on number fifteen, happens instantly after the zap, radiation seems gentle, as does everything: friends, the air, the expectations I impose on myself. Nothing hurts, with the exception of a new radiation guy, John, pimply and so young he probably just graduated from moving cars up and down on another kind of hydraulic lift. He scolds me for sitting up when I am still five feet up in the air, before the bed is all the way back down to floor level. I say that I won't jump. He says the mattress might lurch and that I could slide off and that his supervisor would give it to him and that he's thinking about my safety. And yours, I retort. I am not a Toyota, I say to myself.

Spots. Her Baldness is now going around unhatted on a regular basis and has passed, except for that spot in the back where hair goes first on men, into a woman with very very very short hair, mainly silver and extremely soft. This woman is getting a lot of pats. Her pate is as delicious as puppy tummy, except when she is having a hot flash, which she does quite often these days, instant menopause being another side effect of chemo, though one of the benefits of chemo, in retrospect, is that a woman of my age finishes up the perimenopause grind—headaches, fatigue, mood swings, etc.—without really noticing. It's like hitting your finger with a hammer to cure a headache.

Anyway. Some people are extremely polite and ask to pat. Other people, especially at a big fiftieth for a colleague that Her Baldness just attended, pat without asking, including people she has never met or only just met, these latter categories including some total babes. There is something restorative about having the hand of an unknown blonde twenty something stroke your head while she tells you that you look like Sigourney Weaver and your true love to whom you are deeply and forever committed looks on not minding. HB doesn't mind pats AT ALL, just for the record, as it makes her feel as much like a rock star, or a puppy, as she is ever likely to feel. These are quite different kinds of love, and she has issues about love, but she is delighted to have all kinds of love, also for the record. Screw her issues. Her friends and acquaintances tell her she looks beautiful, for which she is grateful. Most people say her head is perfectly shaped.

Almost all women and most of the men then add something like, I could never shave my head because I have a weird place, or because I have a bad place, or because I have a funny place. This place is usually described as flat though on a few occasions it has been specifically described as a bump. Invariably, when HB's interviewees touch the place they dislike, which they do uncertainly and tentatively, the spot is located slightly below the crown, that is, right between the eyes in the back of the head. When HB touches the place, through the hair that covers it, and no she doesn't always ask, it has been, with one exception attributable to physical trauma, of a roundness and smoothness perfectly and absolutely consistent with the curvature of the rest of the person's head. It is, however, a place the person themselves cannot easily see, even with the help of a mirror. HB thinks she is onto something really big here. She thinks she has found a place demonstrably more elusive and possibly more deadly by far than either of the poles, a place that was close to home after all, a place that has everything to do with desire and shame and terror and guilt and extreme vulnerability. HB thinks she has found the mortality pressure point. It's the place to touch for reassurance when you are feeling really glad it's not you that has cancer. There's nothing wrong with having this place or touching this place. Everyone has it. Everyone does it. It's like masturbating, or maybe like learning how to have good sex. It's often easier to find the most interesting place while you're looking at someone else's.

Staging. Breast cancer is organized by degrees of seriousness that determine the severity and the permutation of the slash, poison and burn regimen, to borrow Susan Love's phrase. Stage one is a tumor under 2 centimeters with no lymph nodes. Stage two is a small tumor with positive lymph nodes, a tumor between 2 and 5 centimeters with either positive or negative lymph nodes, or a tumor larger than 5 centimeters with negative lymph nodes. Stage 3 is a tumor bigger than the ones we have been talking about with positive lymph nodes. Stage 4 is a tumor that has metastasized to other parts of the body, like bones or lungs or liver. Not all of the people in my support group have breast cancer, and other cancers are staged differently, but using this rough system, at least four of my peers have attained a higher stage than I. Two of them, to my knowledge, have terminal diagnoses and I think another also does but isn't saying so and another one, unfortunately but not coincidentally the one who is the hardest to like, may have put herself in their company because she has missed more chemo appointments than anyone can count. We no longer bother to ask her why or attempt to persuade her of the wisdom of going.

Medical service providers often manifest concern about support groups that put people with different cancers, or different stages of cancer, in the same room. They think those with less serious cases might incur additional stress by exposure to fears they do not yet need to have and stress, as we all think we know, is bad for people with cancer. This is particularly true in my support group, where strategies to avoid stress are promoted without question, though is not clear whether avoiding stress cures the disease or merely makes one feel better on the way out. The difference is, at any rate, academic. I know I am flirting with death. I use the support group to ensure that I can flirt without being seduced because I believe I can hold out for a good long time. I don't know whether I suffer more stress as a result, or whether those with more advanced stages of cancer suffer more stress because of me.

WEDNESDAY | OCTOBER 18, 2000

Diarrhea this morning. Dark green and oily. Not my day to see the doctor and I cannot bear to stand in the middle of the waiting room, holding it in, and plead my case to the nurse. Stomach hurts on the right side. Scaly patches on my elbows and legs. Today's preparation for the last nine radiations, the booster beam. A pie-shaped wedge on my right tit, outlined in lead wire for The Sim.

THURSDAY | OCTOBER 19, 2000

Green shit, day two. Why go to an event with a huge crowd and eat spinach quiche cooked years before? HB won't talk about disgusting stuff in public. Her Baldness is pulling her punches.

FRIDAY | OCTOBER 20, 2000

Green shit, day three. Stand in the middle of Cedars waiting room doing my best. I find the nurse who finds a doctor. Blood count is tested. Don't get dehydrated, drink even if you don't eat, come into the clinic over the weekend if it gets worse. Kim and I fight over the size of rice grains, whether short- or long-grained brown is better. I buy short, she prefers long.

SATURDAY | OCTOBER 21, 2000

IN A MESSAGE DATED 10/21/00 SUSANC WRITES: i hope you are well and resting. i miss you at school and i hope you get better soon.

THURSDAY | OCTOBER 26, 2000

I have a bladder infection. Also shooting pains down my right arm. Not to worry, the nerve is re-generating. I need a cancer vacation.

Group. Suzie woke coughing blood. Was it fresh? asks Evelyn. Tom has gained 13 pounds.

MONDAY | OCTOBER 30, 2000

IN A MESSAGE DATED 10/30/00 CSELL WRITES: Renee told me about your breast cancer diagnosis and treatment. I'm so sorry to hear of this. Realizing there may not be much that I can do or that you would wish me to do, know that I am holding you in my thoughts. And know that I would be happy to help in any way I can.

TUESDAY | OCTOBER 31, 2000

Kim in Miami. Arm no better.

IN A MESSAGE DATED 10/31/00 CBLORD@UCI.EDU WRITES TO UNDISCLOSED RECIPIENTS: SUBJECT: HER BALDNESS TRIES TO ABDICATE

Her Baldness, when she runs her hand over her head, feels stuff up there. Loft. Texture. Nap. Resistance. Not just puppy tummy but in a few places more like recently shorn terrier. Her Baldness tries to be as honest as a drag queen can be, which is pretty fucking honest when the circumstances are right and deadly, when she's in the zone. Her Baldness has therefore been anticipating turning in her handicapped windshield tag, so to speak, now that there's fuzz, renouncing the title or at least turning it over to the next lucky person who gets the gift of cancer.

Turns out that it ain't so easy to resign. Two weeks ago I drove to Irvine, or rather I was graciously and generously driven down by Yong Soon and Allan and driven back by Annie, as I wasn't so sure about the fatigue level and the 5 south to the 605 south to the 405 south to the 73 south commute that is an hour on the good days. I went to see a colleague in women's studies who had been diagnosed with ovarian cancer this summer, now going through six rounds of chemo, and to attend the opening of the Beall Center (the UC Irvine art gallery revamped as a high tech media center). I needed a little excitement and I wanted to be present at whatever arts glamour could happen for a night behind the orange curtain and I wanted to support the gallery director and my colleagues who had curated the show if not exactly to

OCTOBER 2000 | 146

see the show itself because it involved a level of attention to computer screens that I didn't want to muster on opening night.

Her Hirsuteness wanted people to know she wasn't dead yet, and had therefore planned an unannounced appearance at her place of employment. She got moderately dressed up in various black things from Barneys. She thought she might conceivably be taken for His Hersuitness but she looked quite fine as him, or her, and it didn't much matter to her either way. Champagne and donated hors d'oeuvres (e.g., stuffed mushrooms, raw tuna, eclairs, jello) outside the gallery. HB mingled. Many many many many hugs. Also, over and over and over again, shocked faces trying to rein it in, or to connect the phrase "Catherine has breast cancer" with the woman standing before them. Cancer improves the peripheral vision. A certain amount of speechlessness. Dominant reaction: You look FABULOUS bald. Maybe it was the lighting. I'm not bald, HB said, at least forty times. You can get away with being bald, said a student. You have beautiful bone structure. Welcome to the world of cool bald people, said a colleague. I'm not bald, Robert, said Her Baldness. YOU are.

But if hair has anything to do with democracy, I didn't have hair, even while making jokes at my own expense about never, not ever, wanting long hair again or in fact any hair longer than this or about the insanity of going through so much to arrive at an advanced haircut, or about the tremendous sums I allegedly save on hair products. Her Baldness was the corpse sitting up in the coffin in a bad old movie. Nobody could see her or hear a word she said because she shook them up and meanwhile she was trying to put them at their ease by making jokes about the pallor of her complexion. The abdication was a flop. Her Baldness couldn't climb out of the fucking coffin. She was stared through by no less than two associate deans. Her head might as well have been made of clear crystal. She was wrecking their party. Her sweetest audience was insignificant staff members and her students. (Was this always true? and if so should I rethink my fantasies of departure from the infomercial that is teaching?) They gave her huge hugs and said exactly what she wanted to hear: we miss you, we want you to come back, it's so dead here without you, you can't IMAGINE what we have to sit through these days, it's so boring. HB also ran into a certain number of colleagues to whom she hadn't spoken since her diagnosis. Hugs of varying strengths. Air kisses. Eddies of hot air. How

ARE you? How have you been? I meant to send you a card, but time got away from me.

A rant, then, probably ill-advised and certainly parenthetical and admittedly ill-tempered. These are people with whom I've had friendly relations. I've helped some of them get jobs and keep jobs. I ask about their pets and their boyfriends and their girlfriends and their mothers and fathers. I go to their shows. Phone too heavy? Post office too far away? Time flies when you're having fun. Killing time. Time on your hands. Making time. Finding time. Passing time. Buying time. I ran out of time. Time got away from me. The summer was over before I knew it. Cancer people talk about how some people let you down, about how most people don't want to hear what's actually going on, and how some of the people you think will be there simply evaporate. Some cancer people say they don't mind, they don't harbor resentment, they adjust their expectations. Though I've made considerable progress, I'm not there and I don't believe any human being with whom I myself actually am acquainted is at such an advanced state of detachment. I am learning to have deep gratitude for what comes my way from unexpected quarters, and there has been much of that. But FYI in HB's Department of Etiquette, for those of you who have friends who know someone who is sick and are wondering whether to send a card or wondering what to do or wondering whether a phone call would be an intrusion—it isn't. It doesn't matter if you don't know exactly what to say. Facing your own mortality is a lonely thing, and it is one of the times, except perhaps at the very end, when people do not want to be alone. Even though you cannot really be there with someone, and even though you cannot face their mortality for them, or take the necessity of facing their own mortality away from them, small and even perhaps old-fashioned social gestures help.

On the other hand, not only does Miss Manners have the tendency to go off on longwinded diatribes, Miss Manners is a fraud. I bitch in spite of, and perhaps because, I've failed people in the past out of my own fear, my own disgust, my own out-and-out repulsion at their sickness and pain. I've stared and backed off and distanced myself from what I perceived to be needs that would overwhelm me, afraid to be drowned in a sea where someone else is going under. I want people to show a compassion for me that I haven't shown to others. Now that I have the knowledge to be compassionate, it's too late for them, if not exactly for me. This is why, I confess, I went to see that colleague in her third round of chemo. We have been close only in principle. I have been a little dismissive of her as an old fashioned seventies sort of lesbian. Now I note how very little hair she has left, and I see her eyes, which happen to be a light blue. We do the slow flirtation of cancer people. When she goes out, she wears a hat to cover her baldness because she doesn't want to scare people. Both of us have had friends who died. Neither of us got it until now. What stage? Lymph nodes? Second opinions? Side effects? Chemo brain? Have some of your colleagues just disappeared?

We chuckle at our fascination with death. We mention our partners' difficulty speaking of the subject. And indeed, when her partner walks into the house, we change subjects in mid-sentence. There's a book called *How to Die*, my colleague whispers to me as we say goodbye, and she lends me other classics: *Cancer in Two Voices*, by Sandra Butler and Barbara Rosenblum, *The Red Devil: A Memoir About Beating the Odds*, by Katherine Russell Rich, *February Light: A Love Letter to the Seasons During a Year of Cancer and Recovery*, by Heather Trexler Remoff, and *Seeing the Crab: A Memoir of Dying Before I Do*, by Christina Middlebrook.

As Kim is not home when I get back, I binge. Two of the authors are still with us, two aren't. When Kim returns I am satiated and remorseful. She makes an intervention. STOP IT, she says. Put them away. Take a vacation. We develop a list of the similarities between cancer books and porn. Here it is. Feel free to add yours.

Other people do it better.
There is a certain amount of shame attached to getting aroused.
One way or another, you pay for it.
You lose bodily fluids.
You're relieved it isn't actually you.
As much as you hope to escape your bodily predicament, there's a little
    too much reality involved.
It can mess up your relationship.

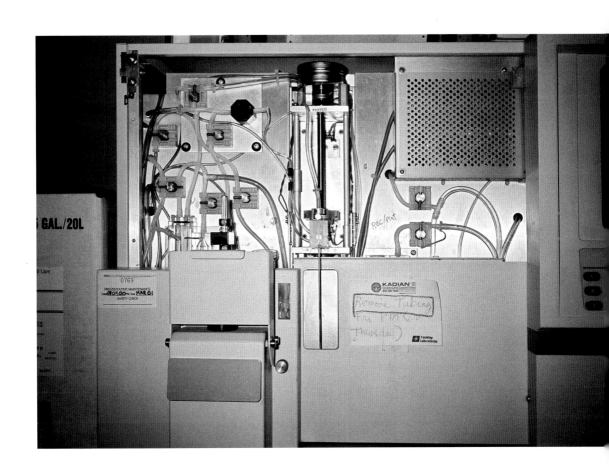

NOVEMBER | 2000

THURSDAY | NOVEMBER 2, 2000

IN A MESSAGE DATED
11/2/00 WHYRAIN WRITES:
Both generate fascination and secrecy.
Really looking forward to Thanksgiving. Ordering the bird today.

FRIDAY | NOVEMBER 3, 2000

IN A MESSAGE DATED
11/3/00 AVEST WRITES:
It doesn't matter how out of date the material is.
It gets you focused, temporarily eliminating other preoccupations.

IN A MESSAGE DATED
11/3/00 ANNEJUN WRITES:
chris said he felt badly about calling you baldy. i was supposed to get
mine chopped this a.m. but the appt got cancelled.

IN A MESSAGE DATED
11/3/00 CBLORD@UCI.EDU
WRITES TO ANNEJUN:
i knew baldy was an endearment.

SATURDAY | NOVEMBER 4, 2000

I used to like the attention being given to the site of the trouble, but now it itches and offends.

MONDAY | NOVEMBER 6, 2000

IN A MESSAGE DATED
11/6/00 LORRGRAD WRITES:
Your missives always astounded me, they were so full of evidences of
love, of a life that was full and had built a community of people to
reach out to. I couldn't imagine it. But I should have known better,
I guess. We always need the right kind of love, and that's always scarcer
than we need.

Three more zaps. Julia Marie gives up. I have gobs of anesthesia in my brain, she says, between the lobes. She can't get anywhere with the brandy but I float to deep greens and blues. Jodie the physical therapist calls about the lymphedema sleeve. It must be fitted specially. Wear it on the plane. If you notice your hand looks young, put it on. Take antibiotics immediately if you see your hand turning red.

Gore concedes.

Al Gore ahead after all. Kim to New York. Buy the lymphedema sleeve. You don't want to be the one that has cancer. You want people there with you. I have felt held by the medical routine and am spinning into orbit at the idea of being completely on my own.

IN A MESSAGE DATED 11/9/00 DEWDROP2U WRITES: Black Barney's. shit woman, you must have looked hot!!! Earthlink lost my email and I HATE THEM!!!!!

First day without something to do every day. Bush sliding.

Group. Dotcom John with the brain tumor thinks angioplastic drugs are the future. He is investing heavily in the company which produces them.

IN A MESSAGE DATED 11/14/00 CBLORD@UCI.EDU WRITES TO UNDISCLOSED RECIPIENTS: SUBJECT: HER BALDNESS BIDS FAREWELL TO PLANET CANCER Her Baldness graduated from radiation on Thursday last, November 9, 2000, at 12.04 p.m., just before Mrs. Thelma Holden and just after Ms. Judy Shapiro. Her Baldness received her graduation certificate, signed and annotated by Darrin and Joanie (KEEP SMILING!!!!) while she was sitting up on the gurney struggling back into her shirt. When Her Baldness left Room 25—which is to be found in the basement of Planet Cancer if you go through the door to the left of the reception desk, then take a left at the Rothko poster and the first right after the second O'Keeffe, directly opposite the Van Goghs—Her Baldness found Mrs.

Holden, who is about seventy five and has lung cancer and a brain tumor and the longest false eyelashes Her Baldness has ever seen, waiting by herself in the hallway in her wheelchair. Mrs. Holden plans to decline the chemo her doctors are trying to persuade her to undertake. Her sister died two weeks ago, the day after *her* first chemo, of kidney failure. Mrs. Holden feels weak and has in mind quality of life. We kissed goodbye and wished each other serenity.

Her Baldness also said goodbye to Mrs. Holden's daughter Gail and to Judy Shapiro, who went through radiation on her other breast eleven years ago and plans to frame her new graduation certificate next to the first one. Judy wishes Her Baldness a long remission, reminding her that you're not cured of cancer until you die of something else. Then Her Baldness drove her burned and itchy right breast back home in an odd state of exhilaration not noticing the traffic or the potholes or the road construction but instead the light and the clear sky and the colors of the signs on shops and fell asleep next to her cat Chloe watching George Bush's lead drop down and down but probably not far enough.

In truth, Her Baldness does not deserve the title these days, but she doesn't plan to give it up. She earned it, like being Dominican or being a dyke. Whether she lives in the United States or checks out the occasional male body or has hair, she retains her titles. She's quite Gertrude Stein from the Roman emperor period, except for a little astroturf on top and wisps that need a bit of trimming at the back of the neck. After she got home from radiation Her Baldness rummaged in the bathroom cabinet behind the leftover baking soda and epsom salts. She got out half a tube of the moulding mud she had gotten in New York five months ago in a state of neurosis and terror and put it on the longer hairs that are becoming flyaway as some of them, but only some of them, are an inch long.

Her Baldness no longer jumps at her reflection in the mirror. She no longer wonders about the transparency of her hair under certain lights. She no longer worries about patches showing through even though at the back of her neck, where she was surprised by a birthmark, it's pretty thin. She doesn't care. She no longer looks pale. Other people, mostly young, with very short hair or no hair, smile at her. She likes thinking that perhaps it's because she's finally joined the secret society of the ultra cool but perhaps it's just that her face is now visible and it wasn't before. She likes having a face. She likes the nakedness of it. She likes being mistaken for a guy. She likes being ambiguous. She likes her hair gray with very little black. She doesn't want any more chemicals near her skin. She doesn't care if she looks older and she doesn't think she does and anyway she hopes she's lucky enough to have the option of looking older. She doesn't care that her ears stick out. She's over that legacy from her grandfather. She's over hiding. She doesn't care if her tummy rolls come back. She sees them now as a buffer in times of need and she recognizes that she cannot predict times of need.

She doesn't cry when she tells people she has cancer, or not as often, though in truth there are people she still needs to tell and she hasn't faced that yet. And yes, she tells people she has cancer. She has arrived at an amused detachment when she hears things like, "So, what's the prognosis?" or, "Are you optimistic?" or, "Well, I'm really sorry to hear the news but you LOOK fabulous." She doesn't much mind when she sees people trying to figure out whether she actually is going to get better or whether she's on her way out in a state of highly articulated denial. She's happy to have paddled a bit in the River Styx and to be toweling off on this side though she has glimpsed the other bank and knows that the light plays tricks on you, especially over water, and it's hard to tell just how far away the other bank is and whether the undertow is carrying you there or back or whether the earth you thought was solid is in fact moving. She's content to be warm and dry and alive and sitting at her computer.

She went to her support group last week. Glenda's right arm is entirely bandaged. She lifted too many weights and she has lymphedema. Naturally she brought information and naturally Doris went off to xerox it. No weights above 15 pounds, no needles, cuts, insect bites, animal bites or bruises. No injections in that arm. Get a sleeve. A medical emergency bracelet is available. The group has enlarged in the last month or so, though some of the newcomers have been one night stands. There's Laura (metastasized colon, inoperable), Mary (squamous cell vaginal), John (brain), Paul (pancreatic, inoperable), Marisol (bilateral stage 2 breast) and Albert (metastasized colon 3B, inoperable). The men bond. "How big is yours?" The women giggle.

Albert, an orthopedic surgeon in his late sixties, spending the night of his twenty fifth wedding anniversary in his first cancer support group, just a month into chemo and wearing a baseball cap, asked HB how long it had taken her hair to grow back. Two months after the last chemo, she explained, like a veteran, and adds that not everyone agrees that it has grown back. Some people still congratulate me on how good I look bald, which goes to show that having hair is an entirely subjective state, and hair doesn't matter that much anyway. HB was astonished to find herself explaining these things to a surgeon, someone who has presumably seen a lot of death and whom she supposed to be wise in all things, and to boot a man, who, rather than being accustomed to baldness or the idea of baldness because of being a man, seemed suddenly vulnerable and indeed ashamed of his sickness when the group teased him into raising his baseball cap a few inches off his head to check out his bald pate. He held his cap in the air for a few seconds, then replaced it and hung his head. I used to have a full head of hair, he said. It was the worst day of my life when it all began to come out. It was worse than getting the diagnosis. You look wonderful, said HB. Your head is perfect. Hair is only hair. Yeah, said John, the day all my hair fell out in the shower was worse than getting a bone marrow aspiration. So. Live and learn. Essentialism rears its ugly head right in front of Her Baldness, who thought she was over that piece of intellectual work, even though she herself could be found this last summer wide awake in the middle of the night watching infomercials about hair transplants.

And a few reminiscences about radiation, while HB still has a hot pink pie-shaped itchy peeling wedge on her right breast which unfortunately does not yet feel like MY right breast. The worst isn't the burn or the itch or the chore of having to be in the same place at the same time every day, something I had arranged my entire life to avoid, but the way you become attached to your captors, the way soft and malleable flesh grows accustomed to being rolled and twisted and jiggled into position by twenty-year-old guys lining up their red laser lines with your tattoo dots to shoot down the target which just happens to be a heavily eroticized part of your queer and female body. Radiation, unlike mammography, is apparently a guy thing: what needs to be lifted on and off a horizontal gurney is often dead weight. It's true that radiation fatigue doesn't feel like much after chemo, but the way radiation grows to occupy more and more space in your life is insidious, altogether too reminiscent of a cancer. By the time you feel the lump, it has already taken over. And when the foreign element has been excised, there's a dent.

The chemo has, in theory, killed any errant cancer cells in my body. The radiation has, according to Dr. Palmer, sterilized my breast, which, after all, not being part of my body, in her words, could have been amputated. My body could not tolerate any more of either chemo or radiation and in addition further treatment would not be effective, statistically and of course financially speaking. Further chemo wouldn't improve my chances sufficiently to make it worthwhile for my insurance company to pay. Therefore nothing is now being done to my body. What's left of my immune system is on its own. So is my paranoia.

I begin to make doctors' appointments: the ovarian ultrasound and Ca125 blood test, the colonoscopy, the oncologist to ask about other blood marker tests for tumors, the visit to the dermatologist to check on those moles, the compression sleeve to protect my right arm against lymphedema when I fly and thus from the subsequent "sometimes tragic" infections described in the brochure sent to me by the physical therapist, the dentist to get my teeth cleaned now that my blood count is back in the normal range, even the ophthalmologist to get a prescription for new glasses. This is what people mean when they opine about taking responsibility for one's health. This is what support group rhetoric describes as being a proactive consumer of traditional medicine. HB knows better. It's not safe to say goodbye to the kidnappers. When they say the cure for cancer has not yet been discovered, they mean that when you catch it, you have it for the rest of your life.

THURSDAY | NOVEMBER 16, 2000

IN A MESSAGE DATED 11/16/00 LCRUX WRITES:

I don't know how you are now, but I hope that all is well and that you are indeed recovering, recovered, healed, healing—all of it. Am in love big time. Met Ms. Right and luckily for me she feels similarly.

IN A MESSAGE DATED 11/16/00 GENAB WRITES:

BE BEAUTIFUL—even if death may be 'round the corner. It really is for ALL of US: nobody knows who'll be going OUT next.

IN A MESSAGE DATED 11/16/00 CSELL WRITES:

When the disease claims your body, then the doctors back up that claim with their own. When all you can claim as your own is your mind and your emotions, is it a declaration of freedom to give those away boldly to whomever you wish?

Gynecologist cannot find my ovaries. Chemo has withered them.

IN A MESSAGE DATED
11/18/00 CBLORD@UCI.EDU
WRITES TO UNDISCLOSED
RECIPIENTS:

SUBJECT: WOMAN FAKES CANCER FOR CASH, GETS PROBATION

BOSTON—A woman who pretended to have cancer and bilked friends, neighbors and family members out of more than $43,000 was sentenced to two years' probation.

Kristen Clougherty, 25, pleaded guilty to larceny and was ordered to repay the money and perform 300 hours of community service. She used the money for breast enlargement surgery, a new car and hotel stays, prosecutors said.   *Los Angeles Times*, Nov. 2, 2000

Christyne L. in Los Feliz pastry shop. Catherine, what's with the hair? I explain. Oh well. Whatever. You look fabulous. She talks of all the money she has raised for her dance department.

We fly to New York for Thanksgiving. I am unremarkable on the street, even in my brother's hair.

Back home. Sir in the bank. She can help you now, sir. At first I don't realize I am being addressed, and then, when the woman repeats it, sir, over here, sir, hello, sir, I pretend not to hear. When she stops saying sir, I go over to her. My own little behavioral modification program. I can tell by her fixed stare and her unwavering smile that she is embarrassed, but she does not apologize.

Kim exhausted. Beginning to waffle on Paris and Spain. I feel unable to make or to count on plans with her. Right now I need to count on things. Shut down because I can't yet afford to let go.

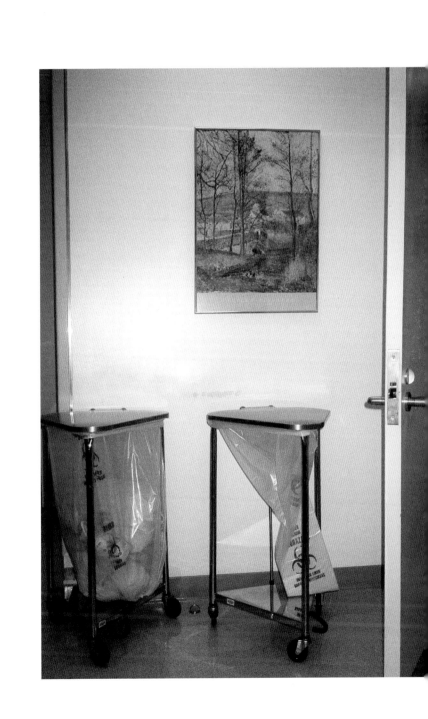

DECEMBER | 2000

Kaucilya's party. Huge hugs from Ellen B., who has been through it. Tears run down my cheeks. I'm just making the most of every precious moment, she says, full of energy and life.

I feel so tired.

Back from visiting my mother in Iowa on Sunday, just missing a monster blizzard. Afterwards flat out for a few days.

Sometimes you need to tell a child what they want isn't good for them, says the shrink. I think you're nuts to go to Paris.

When Felix and Ross were sick, Felix pushed himself to go to Paris with Ross so that they could do everything they wanted to do in their lives before Ross died. They both knew Ross would go first. Felix is dead now.

IN A MESSAGE DATED 12/15/00 CBLORD@UCI.EDU WRITES TO UNDISCLOSED RECIPIENTS:

SUBJECT: NOTES ON SOME THINGS BEGINNING WITH T

Talk. I have ceased to do so in my support group, which is now about eight women and four men. I attribute to the latter the fact that conversation has shifted from feelings to fish stories about chemo recipes, weight loss and staging. The facilitator seems incapable of bringing the talk back round. In fact, she flirts girlishly with Tom, the man most responsible for reducing all conversation to shop talk. Sorry to hear they couldn't operate on yours, buddy, OR, yeah, yeah, I'm on Gemzar too. How about that nausea? Yeah, and how about that numbness in the old fingers? The men might as well be swapping tales of RAM or engine oil. At our last meeting, much too near the group hug at the end to take issue, Tom told me that he liked me better without what he referred to as my black skating cap. "I knew there was a pretty lady under there," he announced. The facilitator waited to see which part of this sentence would set me off. Lecture on feminism to a dying old man whose pretty young wife in the next room cooks whatever will tempt him because he himself doesn't know how to boil water and certainly isn't going to learn now that time is running out? Suggest that Tom has problems with my masculinity? And my femininity? Not me.

Taste. Famous woman artist of psychoanalytic proclivities whose own hairstyle, unchanged for thirty years, has been the subject of much off-the-record art world speculation as to its structural engineering and signification: Well, Catherine, I suppose when a woman gets to be a certain age, cutting it off is one option.

Taxonomy. Ten years ago, or four years ago, or two years ago, depending on which school of military history one prefers, something landed in my body and set up camp, seizing rich natural resources and diverting them to its own greater glory. Before anyone noticed, the colony had taken the shape of an island, roughly twice as long as it was wide, of an irregular surface. Folded ridges of tissue. No normal terrain. A diffuse gritty mass. I was born there. What is your cancer trying to teach you? That's the question people want answered. Given the fact that you are being punished, of what crime are you guilty?

Tears. In group, Albert the orthopedic surgeon asks whether people cry. All the men say yes, and then all the women. Albert is taking Adriamycin, Cytoxan and Prednizone. He has another three months to go. He can't stop crying. He cries over TV commercials. He cries reading magazines. I ask him if he is ashamed of being sick, if he feels like more of a failure than the rest of us because he is a doctor. No. He has treated so many sick people in his life that he never believed it couldn't happen to him. He has made a Christmas card with a photo of his family every year of his married life but this year, when he cannot take his hat off for more than a few seconds, he cannot imagine posing for the photograph. We persuade him otherwise, we hope. Tom talks about his temper. He loses it with his wife again and again. She yells back. As he speaks his face crumples and he cannot get the words out.

Tenderness. I've had a chemical peel. Skin, heart, mind, memory have been rubbed thin. I cry, anywhere, anytime, at any sign of affection or compassion, but particularly when it comes from other women who have been through this, the so-called survivors. When I catch their eyes scanning me for the signs of the place they themselves used to inhabit, I lose it. Your eyebrows grew back, said Annetta. She warns me to watch out for depression. It is common when they stop doing things to you and you have to pick up the pieces of your life. I've not wanted to let go because the way to get through a present that consists of pain and fear is to hold it together, to resist anything that would spark a connection between the surface of my body and the currents flowing inside. Under the circumstances, touch has ranged from abrasive to terrifying. Finally, a few Sundays ago, no compelling reason to rise, sunshine outside, I kiss Kim. She takes her sweet time. I don't care where we go or when and so we do.

Testaments. I was in the middle of chemo and I wanted to be sure Kim could unplug me if push came to shove. I was in more of a hurry to take care of this piece of business than she. I didn't count on our dyke lawyer's vacations, or her grandchildren, or her need to attend the Democratic convention, not to mention our inability to decide where the money should go if we both died together in a plane crash and the number of phone calls required to get a notary and witnesses together with two clients and one lawyer in a conference room. We now have in our possession two manila envelopes, one labeled "Kim's documents" and the other, "Catherine's documents." They contain our wills and our durable health care power of attorneys. We are both registered, at our respective places of employment, as domestic partners. I visit the University of California benefits counselor to inquire into disability and possible retirement. You have to decide on your life expectancy, the counselor explains. If you only plan to live ten years, you would be all right. If you live longer, you will be poor. How long do you think you will live? They used to test for witches by holding obstreperous women under water. If the woman drowned, you knew she was innocent.

Tests. I've passed Ca125, the blood test marker for ovarian cancer, as well as a color ultrasound for the same thing. Your ovaries are there and they are homogenous, said the specialist to whom I had been referred by my gynecologist when she was unable to find them on her little black and white monitor. He meant that as a compliment. I didn't clear the bloodletting section of the exam. When the nurse went to put a band aid on the vein in my hand afterwards, blood had ballooned into a bulge the size of a grape. I TOLD you to apply pressure, she said, pushing the grape flat. Flooded with fear, I burst into tears. It's not serious, she said. It will be OK. All you'll get is a bruise. Health care providers are divided into those who understand how thin-skinned cancer patients are and those who do not.

Texture. Three months out of chemo, it's past puppy tummy but nothing to run the fingers through. It has thickness, far more than it had in my long-haired days. It has traction. It has eddies and backwaters and rapids. It's a salt marsh. It's a cowlick patch. It is exactly the hair of my brother who died a stupid death at seventeen. I comb it to the side, as Robert did. I make circles in it with my forefinger, then calm the turbulence. These are my brother's gestures. My mother and my sister are the only people in the world who could possibly attest to this reincarnation. They don't live in Los Angeles. They haven't seen this stage. They do not call up my brother the same way I do. That I have regrown my brother's hair is my secret. It affords me the calm to register pleasure when I am called sir.

Thanksgiving. When Kim and I visited New York in September, between chemo and radiation, I happened to mention to Yvonne that we would probably come to New York after everything was over. You're both invited to Thanksgiving, she said immediately. In addition to the organic turkey and the brussels sprouts and mashed potatoes and pear parsnip puree and three kinds of pie, it was the first time in five months that I had enough up there not to be obliged to talk about breast cancer in a group of people. Perhaps everyone knew, perhaps not, but the relief was in not having to explain or reassure or amuse or to still the pain that flicks across other people's faces, and to be unsure whether the pain is their pain or a reflection of the pain on my own face. It is liberatory to speak of things other than cancer. This is related to being able to walk down the street, or into a store, or a restaurant, without catching out of the corner of my eye the movement of heads as they turn and then turn again, rapidly, lest they be caught staring at a sick woman. Her Baldness is fading into the woodwork, which is not coextensive with the closet. She talked with the nice fag selling her an earring about the practical difficulties of having a short haircut in winter. She did not feel obliged to share with him the fact that he was, technically, the only one with a haircut. She was mistaken by her friend John Mason Kirby, while she sat in a restaurant awaiting his arrival, for a middle aged man cruising him. She is regularly checked out by dykes on the street.

Thick. People used to say that of my mother's hair when she was young and a beauty and her hair fell in auburn waves to her shoulders. When I went to see her at the beginning of December, her hair was completely white. For the first time I could see through to the pink of her scalp. My mother was relieved to see me, vastly relieved, and relieved to see me walking and strong. Your hair's fine, she announced. I like it. But it would also look nice a little longer. Why do you keep pulling on it? It's a habit, I explain, defensively. It's left over from chemo. I'm testing to see if it's still attached. My mother reads biographies to tally the obstacles others have overcome. She isn't particularly interested in either motivation or failure. It is easier for her to express remorse for a Boer trunk she left behind when she moved to the U.S. than it is to speculate about her marriage to the drunken husband she followed there. Together, we negotiate fatigue. I can't do everything, she says, but I can do some things.

Time. This is the only thing that will convince you that you have your life back, says the oncologist. Your hair comes back a lot faster than your head.

Tint. As a child I was fascinated with stories in which someone's hair turned white overnight because of sorrow or pain or sickness. I badly wanted to meet such a person to confirm the truth of the stories. I didn't imagine speaking with them, for I was much too shy a child to meet a stranger and ask them questions, but I wanted at least to see such a person so that I could know the stories were true. I wanted to know someone whose pain had been stamped upon the surface of their body so that all could corroborate it. In July, my hair was brown with a lot of gray. Now, in December, it is completely and definitively gray. No brown at all. I am bemused when other people, particularly women, express sympathy. (You must be very happy to have it back. But it's gray.) I like the look of my hair. I prefer having gray hair to no hair. I do not want to admit that my body has registered an enormous change. I do not want to admit that hair dries up, thins, and loses pigmentation as a result of aging. I cry in my shrink's office when she asks me how I feel about going gray because there was no going.

Tiredness. The euphoria of being done with it all lasted two weeks or so. I'm recognizing now that unless I sleep in the afternoon the evening is leaden. The estimates for getting over the need for a nap range from a month to a year. The naps range from thirty minutes to three or four hours. Radiation fatigue is only now catching up with Kim. She was there for everything, saying I can't lose you, you cannot die, everything will be absolutely fine, until even selfish, pigheaded HB believed her. Kim is just now beginning to be able to say to herself that she could have lost me and that she is profoundly tired.

Tits. Yvonne's scar is white and diagonal and runs across her chest up under her arm. Mine, somehow improved by radiation, is barely visible and tiny. The skin of my breast is back to normal. And I have a breast. Yvonne didn't have chemo or radiation. I did.

Tolerance. Now that I am being monitored rather than treated, people think it's time I got over it. When they ask how I am, they want the short answer. I am not in crisis and I am not as interesting as I used to be.

Trash. For the past six and a half years, I have stored some of my former lover's boxes in the garage, along with a little wooden rocking chair, painted red, that her father made for her when she was a child. My former lover has not wished to speak to me, about her possessions or about the end of our ten-year relationship, since I left her. Until she encountered me by chance at a party in October, she expressed no word of sympathy for my diagnosis. This has been a source of pain. After radiation was over, I decided to do something about her possessions. In the boxes were things I believed my former lover ought to have wanted, or that I would have wanted were I in her place, but I am not in her place, she did not respond to my inquiries and I needed to empty my space of her relics. Over the course of a few weeks, I moved the boxes to the trash. I gave the little red rocking chair to the couple who clean the house. They have a new grandchild. My former lover's father was an angry man. The chair has hammer marks on both armrests where he missed the nails.

Treatment. No one is in charge. I press for follow up recommendations and information. I neither want to fall off the grid nor to become a high maintenance body. Your gynecologist will want you to get an ovarian ultrasound, says the radiation oncologist. I will refer you for a bone density scan. You won't really need another mammogram for a year but if you insist upon it you can have one in six months. The gynecologist refers me to the ultrasound lab, and that specialist says I should have an ultrasound at least every six months. You must get an internist, says the gynecologist, and she will want to check your heart as chemo damages the heart. You must also get a colonoscopy. I make the arrangements. We will check your blood every three months, says the oncologist, white and red and hemoglobin as well as liver and calcium. My calendar looks like this. December: dermatologist, dentist (put off due to chemo), check up with oncologist. January: check up with surgeon, radiation oncologist, internist, dermatologist, get colonoscopy. March: blood tests. April: bone density. May: Pap smear, follow-up mammogram. June: ovarian ultrasound, blood tests. I have never had so many doctors' appointments in my life. I'm amortizing those fifty-one years when I ate like a horse, smoked like a chimney, drank like a fish and could still say my health was excellent. Time for the balloon payment. Everyone thinks you're all done when you're over radiation, says Susan S. It's not like that. You're just going into limbo.

Tumor. I've lately removed from the refrigerator door the picture that has been there since the end of last May, when Kim and I received The Diagnosis. I couldn't understand then what it was I was said to have, what Ed the surgeon actually meant when I spoke to him from my car phone stuck in a traffic jam on the 710 and he told me that it was 99 percent certain my fine-needle biopsy was positive and I needed to make immediate arrangements for surgery. I didn't understand what cancer was, or what it did, or how it worked, or how it kills. I knew it was something to fear, but I couldn't picture it in my mind, only on other people's faces.

The photograph on the refrigerator door, ripped from *Harvard Magazine*—which was using it to publicize its latest efforts to stream research revenue in the direction of Cambridge, Massachusetts—was an electron microscope scan of a single cancer cell, dyed magenta and cyan, floating against a black background. It looked like something a nerdy scientist with art pretensions would find beautiful, a round lobed thing with spikes, a pomo blunderbuss, no worse and no better, for all I knew, than the well behaved and productive cells, the good cells, would look if similarly tarted up on glossy paper. Kim and I called it the purple disco ball. For a while I made light of it, with Kim and with everyone else. Even when I tried to imagine tens of thousands, hundreds of thousands, millions and billions of purple disco balls rolling down my veins and multiplying until they clotted in lumps, I couldn't really muster up the aggression to hate the purple disco ball and its friends because it was, after all, only a purple disco ball and its picture was stuck to my refrigerator with an old magnet of the Five Lesbian Brothers. The disco ball was an abstraction and therefore impotent.

I took issue with the military metaphors that surround cancer: war, battle, aggressive measures, forceful intervention, etc. etc. I thought fighting was beneath me, that only people with bad politics and shallow minds cured themselves by turning to battle as a way to find strength. But this fall, when I found the disco ball underneath the various get well cards stuck to the refrigerator with other magnets, I noticed that Kim had crossed it out with a big black X. The more chemo went on the more I came to hate the purple disco ball, or to understand that the relations being negotiated between that abstraction and my body were the cause of my pain, so that I could, in truth, suck some strength out of hating the purple disco ball as something considerably more threatening to my life than bad art, until eventually Kim covered it up with more innocent things, like cards and pictures of other people's babies.

Perhaps the turning point in accepting what I didn't want to accept happened one night in group with Doris, the customs officer. I am coming to understand that she arrives in front of potential audiences with a story to recite, a story that she is prepared to repeat, with conviction, over and over again. Doris describes her various tumors by recourse to food. Some were hardboiled eggs and some were grapes but the main one was the grapefruit that had pushed her uterus back against her spine. Perhaps that night her audience wasn't attentive enough to her ovarian cancer, for Doris reached into her purse and pulled out a picture of her grapefruit, that is to say, the pathologist's picture of her primary tumor. Do you all want to look at it? she asked. Naturally we did and so the picture set off around the circle before the facilitator could think of a rule that would allow her to stop us.

What's that sausage thing? someone asked. It turned out to be Doris's fallopian tube. That decoded, we could pick out the ovary, tiny, and rather like an eyeball, particularly in relation to the tumor, which looked nothing whatsoever like a grapefruit and entirely like a huge bloody lump of gristle. It was getting ready, said Doris, to suck her blood and take over her pelvic cavity. It was ugly. It looked greedy and stubborn and sneaky and stupid enough to grow unchecked for the sake of growing until it put an end to itself by choking the body that was giving it life. It was impossible to imagine containing such a thing with gentle healing thoughts or entertaining the possibility of coexistence with it or adopting any other attitude toward it than an uncompromising desire to exterminate it from the face of the earth by any means necessary.

SATURDAY | DECEMBER 16, 2000

IN A MESSAGE DATED
12/16/00 CSELL WRITES:
I burst into tears reading about Robert's hair.

IN A MESSAGE DATED
12/16/00 WHYRAIN WRITES:
I beg to differ on one not so small matter: you are more interesting than you used to be. Getting back to a life without cancer but full of doctors is like taxes. It's just something you have to do.

TUESDAY | DECEMBER 19, 2000

IN A MESSAGE DATED
12/19/00 CBLORD@UCI.EDU
WRITES TO UNDISCLOSED
RECIPIENTS:
SUBJECT: HER BALDNESS NE VA PAS A PARIS
That's what Kim and I decided last Friday morning, or rather, she left the decision entirely up to me. You are the pitcher and the batter and the catcher and the umpire in this game, she said. She knew that if she decided, I would resist, so she said she would support whatever I decided, no matter what, so I decided and consequently deciding wasn't easy. It hadn't only been Paris. It was Paris then Seville then Granada then Madrid then New York then Los Angeles. When I type this itinerary it sounds ambitious for anyone, much less someone who got cancer, became Her Baldness, and spent six months absorbing into her body substances invented by the military to make genocide more efficient. Kim has been trying for some time now to suggest that a woman who often has to be woken up for dinner and sometimes can barely stay awake to finish the meal and who is currently fighting off a cold might be better off staying at home and resting in order to rebuild her strength. We can go another time, Kim has said, in the spring, or the

summer, when you're better. But of course I resisted and resisted partly because Kim has a tendency not to want to go on vacations when the moment actually comes and partly because in my alcoholic family plans were always being changed or forgotten for reasons entirely out of my control and partly because I don't see why doing geographics is such a bad idea if you can afford it and partly because I have always been able to reach inside myself for a bit more strength and never until now come up so close to empty. Mainly I resisted because I made it through the summer and through the fall by saying to myself and to other people, "It will be over by Christmas and we're going to Paris to celebrate."

Being in Paris would prove that it was indeed all over, and so why not tack on all that fantastic architecture in the south of Spain? Conversely, not getting to Paris at Christmas—even though while I was fighting Kim's desire to cancel I felt a growing dread about airports, airplanes, crowds, rain, cold, etc.—would therefore mean that it wasn't all over and my fatigue was still fatigue. This I did not wish to be true. You're not well enough now, Kim would say. You have huge circles under your eyes. You will be stronger. WAIT. But I don't actually know that I will be stronger, I would say, and besides I want to see the Alhambra before I die. (What am I supposed to say to THAT? Kim asked Dr. Kemeny. For once, Dr. Kemeny didn't have a quick comeback.) If I learned I was going to die, Kim said to me one night as we were dozing off, I would be grateful that I had met you. When YOU get afraid of dying, you make a list of the monuments you haven't seen.

I recognize that Paris is just a symbol and I am aware that Paris is a cold city in many senses of that word and I know it is raining there now and will continue to do so for the foreseeable future but Paris meant Christmas dinner with my ex and her love, a hotel on the Place des Vosges, the dinner of a lifetime at Taillevent, an evening with Annie and her boyfriend Chris, who by chance will be in Paris, a visit to *Olympia* at the Orsay and maybe something sublimely and irresistibly corny like Chartres on Christmas day.

But this is about realizing that my body is not where my mind wants it to be and my body won't go to where my mind wants it to be just because my mind tells it to. Also, when my body feels wiped out my mind goes. Being treated to some peace could be in itself a celebration for this body. Perhaps because I've never been really sick before, I have no image of what it is to heal and no sense of healing as a process that involves a submission to duration rather than imposition of will. Pleasure could be had there. When will I be back to normal? I have asked the experts. The answers vary too much to be useful. In my support group, people say the most frustrating thing is to look well but feel like shit. When they talk about their fatigue, which they all do, their bodies slump, as I am sure mine does.

And then there is Kim. To say that both people in a couple receive the diagnosis is not only to say that both people are exposed to the corrosions of fear and frustration and rage and denial and pain but that these forces wear down both people and that her exhaustion is as real as mine. (For example, she has by my calculations flown 110,000 miles last year, all of that in eight months, as she did not travel when Her Baldness was doing chemo.) So neither of us, in fact, are sorry to cancel the big trip, especially because after we had made our decision we called the most fabulous place in the world on Big Sur and discovered that someone had cancelled twenty minutes before. We shall sit on a high cliff and look over the Pacific at Christmas. The Alhambra will be standing in March, when we now plan to go, and Paris will be there too. There is time. I haven't thrown out the list of monuments.

WEDNESDAY | DECEMBER 20, 2000

IN A MESSAGE DATED 12/20/00 CATGUN WRITES:

okay. i've cried before when i've read HB's writings, but not quite like today's installment. not sure if it's cuz you're "out of the woods" (not doing chemo/radiation/weed killer/military scunge) but/and still not feeling so great that it has a more mundane, and less mysterious, more tangible, less ethereal, more shitty cuz less unreal quality.

IN A MESSAGE DATED 12/20/00 WHYRAIN WRITES:

Airports and timetables and crowds and noise and hotel reservations gone awry and rented cars in narrow cobble-stoned rain-slicked Seville alleys—you really don't need any of that now. Lie around, look at the news, get mad, get incredulous. The Eiffel Tower will still be there. And Olympia's paint no less vibrant. And those cobblestone alleys. And Kim, that exemplary sport, needs a rest.

IN A MESSAGE DATED
12/20/00 SHARHA WRITES: my god, that trip you had planned would have unnerved me. you have to just stay at home and watch movies. do nothing. read trash. play with chloe . . . if i was there i'd make you disgustingly healthy juicer drinks and strap you to your lawn chair with a years supply of mad magazine.

THURSDAY | DECEMBER 21, 2000

IN A MESSAGE DATED
12/21/00 DEBOBR WRITES: Today was mammogram day. The anxious pokings and proddings of every swelling and unexpected pain has pretty much subsided after eight years. But there's still the annual drip feed of terror in the radiologist's waiting room, surrounded and amplified by that of the smocked matrons whose company I keep. Buoyed by the two-word benediction, "no change," I took it as a good omen (even if cost cutting and crushing patient load is the likely reason) that I'd been kicked down the staffing ladder to the nurse practitioner instead of seeing God the Surgeon. I rushed home on wings.

It does get better with time. So does Paris.

IN A MESSAGE DATED
12/21/00 CBLORD@UCI.EDU
WRITES TO UNDISCLOSED
RECIPIENTS: SUBJECT: HER BALDNESS HAS A BRUSH WITH PHILANTHROPY
Two friends on this list wrote to say that they wanted to make a $1,000 donation to the breast cancer organization of my choice. Her Baldness thinks this is a thoughtful and generous idea and so do I, of course, though that said such decisions aren't easy and the four of us have been back and forth about the details. The dilemma is this: give to an organization that would work to solve the problem at the source, or give to an individual who is desperately in need of cash? Teach someone how to farm or give them food? Efficiency or sentiment? Activism or romance? I asked my friends to split the money in two: half to Breast Cancer Action and the other half to Joan Corbin. Breast Cancer Action is easy to check out, and I have spent many hours on their website. Joan Corbin I had never heard of, until, around the same time HB was dithering about her philosophy of philanthropy, I got the following notice on a lesbian artists' list serv to which I belong.

> Joan Corbin, 79, was the art editor of *One Magazine* 1954–1964. *One Magazine* was the publication of One, Inc., an early homosexual rights organization.

Born May 25, 1921 in Armada, Michigan, Joan grew up in Richmond, Michigan. She briefly studied art at Wayne University (Now Wayne State), in Detroit, before moving to California in 1946. Corbin took one course in design at Chouinard where she learned "everything about art." She was the model in some of the nude photographs taken by bisexual photographer Ruth Bernhard.

In August, 2000, Joan Corbin found a lump in one of her breasts. Since September, she has had mammograms, biopsies, and surgery. Dec. 11, 2000, she started bi-lateral radiation. She has lived for many years on a small fixed income and now is seriously in need of financial help.

As it happens, I possess a small stack of *One* ("The Homosexual Magazine"), running from 1953 to 1965. I don't remember where I got them, but I'm irrationally fond of my mini collection. The magazines are tiny, just eight-and-a-half-by-eleven-inch sheets folded and stapled. High seriousness was the order of the day. Most issues feature a statement explaining that the One Institute aimed to deal with homosexuality from "the scientific, historical and critical point of view" and "to sponsor education programs . . . for the aid and benefit of social variants." There are lots of earnest articles about Greeks and Native Americans and long-winded explanations about why homosexuality wasn't a crime against nature. There is fascinating coverage of police entrapment scandals as well as snippets of international news of interest to gays and lesbians (e.g., ENGLAND'S M.P.'S CONSIDER CASTRATION AS CURE FOR SEX OFFENDERS, NUDISTS BATTLE COPS AT ST. TROPEZ, as well as INCOME TAX GUIDE FOR HOMOSEXUALS). *One*'s own groundbreaking legal battles with the U.S. Post Office, which tried in 1954 to stop distribution of the magazine on the charge of obscenity, receive detailed coverage. *One* took the case all the way up to the Supreme Court. In 1958, it won. Nonetheless, every now and then the editors reminded their readers, in case there was any confusion or mislaid desire, that *One* was not an erotic publication.

It wasn't, with the possible exception of the little ads placed by queers who didn't call themselves queers aiming to make a buck. Complete CAST-UR-SELF KIT ($12.95), EL CONFECCION after shave/shower (imparts a singularly soft, warm fragrance — but leaves no bitter denaturants on the skin; $4.70), STRIPPERS' SCHOOLBOOK (learn the proper walk of a lady fully dressed in a gorgeous gown; $1.98), GAY GREETING CARDS (samples 4 for $1), PASS KEY (a stick perfume for men; $2.95), MICHELANGELO'S DAVID (beautifully reproduced in plaster, 23 inches in height, satisfaction guaranteed; $15.95), EXTRA LARGE PECANS (direct from grower in Dixie, 3 pounds $1.95), and BACHELOR'S BUDDY—PORTABLE COOKING UNIT (infrared marvel cooks, brews, toasts and warms; $14.95).

For the obvious reasons, nothing in *One* is what it appears to be. The people who write letters to the editor never use their full names. Instead, it's "Mr. P., Cedar Rapids, Iowa," "Mr. A., Portland, Oregon," "Miss R., Moscow, Idaho," and "Mr. L., Midwest." Fiction is published by people who use an initial instead of a last name or no last name at all. Photo credits go to initials or to names in other countries. Everybody on the masthead, as far as I can tell, was a pseudonym. Betty Perdue (now there's a great fifties club name) was Geraldine Jackson, Sheila Rush was Sten Russell, Allison Hunter was someone called Nancy, Wilna Onthank was sometimes Dawn Fredericks and sometimes Willi Fredericks. And Joan Corbin was Eve Elloree.

According to Jim Kepner (*http://www-lib.usc.edu/~retter/onewomen.html*), in her years at *One*, Joan was at first lovers with Ann Carri Reid, a butch who wanted a stay-at-home wife. Joan left Reid to move in with Sten Russell, and then moved on to a life in the canyons north of Los Angeles with Gingere Blakeley—a horsewoman. Joan's drawings, which she occasionally signed, owe something to Giacometti. The line is delicate, the pen seldom leaves the paper and the figures occupy one dimension more emphatically than the other. They're often doodles, punctuation rather than declaration. The art direction is staid, though there are some noir-ish cover photos of staged pick-up scenes that are priceless. I like the stodginess. It's what happens when people who couldn't talk openly about getting laid put out a zine before there were xerox machines. (Though Betty Perdue admitted to anonymous sex in bushes. Good for her.) It's all about trying to be nice queers and failing, but if it weren't for those queers I wouldn't be here and neither would my young friends who want to make this donation.

As I wrote to them, there are certain coincidences. Lesbians are relatively invisible in (straight) women's breast cancer organizations and lesbians were relatively invisible in the gay male homophile organizations of the 1950s. I have lately been encountering elderly women with cancer and not much money. My mother, who would rather not say words like queer or dyke or lesbian, will be 77 in a few days. Thanks to me, her odds in breast cancer roulette are worse than they used to be. I have breast cancer and I have this little pile of zines. I'm not sure I would have been brave enough to work on such a publication in 1954. Sentiment is not a simple thing.

So here's to Eve Elloree. May her skin not burn too badly and may her technicians be gentle and may she get the rest she needs and may she live to die peacefully in her sleep of something other than cancer.

THURSDAY | DECEMBER 28, 2000

More pubic hair. Depression palpable.

Dinner with Cathy O. What's going on with our friendship? she asks. Sometimes you need to work at friendship, I say. I'm sorry I wasn't there for you, she replies. Why am I the one who weeps?

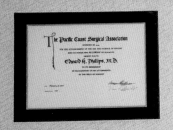

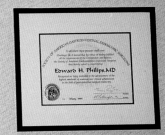

JANUARY | 2001

IN A MESSAGE DATED
1/3/01 SMUHLER WRITES:
Your writing, it transports me to all sorts of nether regions, dark and light. Also it makes me want to ask inappropriate questions—at least in polite company—but only for the best possible reasons. With my friends who have been ill it has always been necessary, ultimately, to throw the niceties out the window. Anyway, Catherine, the long and short of it is I am really proud of you—and I know you don't need me to tell you that—but you have clearly been to Hades and back. Even so, I still hear the same Catherine under all of those words, the same person whom I always admired so much.

Cute haircut, people say now, not you look FABULOUS. Hair all furrows and ridges. It grows out and then changes its mind to head back to my skull.

IN A MESSAGE DATED
1/12/01 CBLORD@UCI.EDU
WRITES TO UNDISCLOSED
RECIPIENTS:
SUBJECT: FIVE THINGS BEGINNING WITH D AND FIVE THINGS BEGINNING WITH F

Decisions. If I had it to do all over again, I would opt for more radical surgery, or so I now think. My breast aches. I try to remove myself from it, to seal it off from my mind. In order for life to return I need to put a barricade between myself and it, between my mind and my body.

Devil, red. This is the street name for Adriamycin. I felt like a hypochondriac for years before the breast cancer: the menopausal woman with mood swings, low energy, headaches, muscle pain, and so on. I complained of these symptoms to my internists again and again. Just wait, they said. Don't worry. As soon as you're through menopause, it will get better. You will stabilize. In *Red Devil*, Katherine Rich describes her symptoms before her breast cancer was diagnosed: fatigue, flu-ish, dragging, generalized muscle aches.

Difficulty. It's not easy to come back. Kim had wanted to make it perfect. My sadness is intractable. In the most beautiful place in the world—three wild turkeys, hawks flying below us in the hot tub, redwood groves, a skyful of stars—we weep. Before we left for Big Sur I noticed that Kim had put away the pictures of me with long brown hair. That woman is dead. Her hair covered her face and of late had owed more and more to the hair colorist to remain competitive in a competitive field. But the woman with long hair, even if she was a girl only in the eyes of her lover, had a body that would open. When we returned, Kim put out a photograph of me sitting on the beach at Malibu, my short haircut two weeks old, before chemo.

Disgust. Tom Hanks spears a crab, breaks off the leg, and pours out brown goo that he can't swallow, no matter how hungry he is. Castaway. He has to invent fire for himself in order to harden goo into matter, to turn it pink, to make it edible. The crab is the sign of repulsion, the creature that walks sideways, balancing on anything, consuming anything, touching, probing, honing its aim, moving in while its eyes look elsewhere. Poking, prodding, silent. Persistent. The cancer sign.

Doodles. After Big Sur, Kim and I went to the Romaine Brooks retrospective at the Berkeley Art Museum. My lesbian art list serv had been full of the show. There had even been a group outing. There was much appreciation of the thousands of colors in Brooks' supposedly monochromatic grays. To me, it was all tinged green. More interesting to talk about how rich Brooks was, and the difference that made, than who she fucked. If she fucked. Her drawings are doodles with the doodle beaten out of them.

First reaction. I don't want to wear a pink ribbon.

Flashes, hot. Do you still have them? my gynecologist asks. Would you like to try something else? She wants to cure them. She is the one who gave me low-dose estrogen in spite of the two grandmothers with breast cancer. The hot flashes are nothing, I say. There are fewer of them, and mainly they happen at night. There are things I have decided no longer need curing. Besides, it now seems to me that hot flashes might have a cleansing function.

Foundation. Blue-clad doctors wait under bright lights next to an operating table at the far end of a swap meet. At the other end, I am trying to undress. The more I try to take off, the more remains. When I get down to my bra, there are four of them. The one next to my skin is Kim's.

Future. Forward bends, in yoga, are supposed to be about the past. The ability to relax in a forward bend is the sign of an advanced student. Backbends are about the future. I have never been able to lift into a backbend without help. When I make the first motions toward the basic poses that will bring me toward the point of imagining a backbend, they are excruciating. My neck, my chest, my belly, the tops of my thighs, even the tops of my insteps are tight. The entire front of my body has contracted in self protection. I try not to take this as an omen but as a reminder that it will take time for the muscles to lengthen. The hair in my armpits has not yet returned, though I have done the Landa steps, all 236 of them, twice now, with many stops to rest. As I work to get stronger, eruptions of the memory of weakness burst through: when my legs felt wobbly climbing down the stairs to my studio, when I would have to sit down on the way from my car to a restaurant, when I couldn't catch my breath because of fear. The act of remembering shifts the contour of the event being remembered. I begin to remember memories.

I am at the bargaining phase, which, I know from hearsay follows anger, denial, and guilt. Next year is way too soon, five years is OK, ten years would be fantastic. Time has shortened. It no longer stretches forward into decades.

Foreigners. When we walk down to Partington's Cove on Big Sur, the late afternoon sun picks out the pampas grass dotting the sides of the hills. It is everywhere: huge, showy, white, sending up great seed-laden heads that blow in the breeze, taking hold, out of scale. Another invasion. They have no business here among the tight, scrubby California natives. They were not here last time I looked. They moved in uninvited. They took hold before anyone realized their presence. Nothing and no one can make them leave now.

SUNDAY | JANUARY 14, 2001

Sylvia and Ed at MOCA yesterday. It was a really busy year and we didn't get the time to call but you look fabulous. We heard from Douglas you looked really beautiful at Thanksgiving. We have been keeping in touch with how you are doing through other people. Thank you, I say. Kim and I are learning to shrug.

WEDNESDAY | JANUARY 17, 2001

IN A MESSAGE DATED 1/17/01 TALA WRITES: you are missed.

MONDAY | JANUARY 22, 2001

IN A MESSAGE DATED 1/22/01 JANECO WRITES: shit, i can't come to your birthday party. just agreed to be in a feminist festival here on campus. the young girls are rising again.

TUESDAY | JANUARY 23, 2001

IN A MESSAGE DATED 1/23/01 MOIRAROT WRITES: it was so lovely to see your email (i know it was a petition—but just seeing your name was such a pleasure.) I know you have been sick, so I just wanted immediately to send you lots of love

THURSDAY | JANUARY 25, 2001

IN A MESSAGE DATED 1/25/01 CBLORD@UCI.EDU WRITES TO UNDISCLOSED RECIPIENTS: SUBJECT: NOTES ON VARIOUS THINGS BEGINNING WITH C AND ONE THING BEGINNING WITH H
Caregivers. According to Bill Moyers, 46% of caregivers are depressed, 43% feel isolated, 70% found new strength, and 36% grew closer to their partner.

Check-ups. Ed Phillips the surgeon has a reputation for good hands. My women doctors say they would go to him if they got breast cancer. He uses the patting-in-a-spiral technique, starting at the outside and working in to the nipple. His hands go on automatic pilot while he chats about other things. He accedes to my desire to remove fluid from the cyst that has formed on the site of the original tumor and fills me with dread whenever my hand finds it. He is unsuccessful. I told you so, he says. It's just plain old rubbery scar tissue. Get another mammogram in March and come and see me in April. Ed was the one who told me the original tumor was probably fine because it didn't feel like a new potato. Nonetheless I decide to trust him.

Dr. Daphne Palmer also gives me a once over. Like Ed, she uses patting-in-a-spiral, but she works from the inside out. I feel fine, at least to her. You will forget this, she says. Now you think of it ten times a day. It'll go down to three or four times a day, and then once or twice a day, and then once or twice a week, and then maybe once or twice a month. Now the cancer is you, but it will eventually become a memory. She is very nice, Daphne Palmer. She knows that I went to Radcliffe, although exactly how she knows this puzzles me, as I am certain I did not tell her, and therefore she always tells me about her daughter who has just started college at Smith and already has a boyfriend.

Dr. Palmer hasn't been through breast cancer herself. Confronted with my pain and fear, she needs to reassure rather than simply to listen. She wants to have something to give, besides radiation, and so she elaborates her reassurances in order to make them true, if only for the moment. Consequently, though I see that she is trying to be nice, I don't trust her. She gives me the Cedars Sinai inaugural pamphlet about lymphedema risks on my right arm (i.e., swelling and infection). I have previously asked her about preventive measures and she prescribed a compression sleeve and antibiotics in case something happens when I'm traveling. If you've had lymph nodes removed you are supposed to treat your arm like a fragile object that has mysteriously attached itself to your body. No cuts, no burns, no extreme heat, no lifting weights. What about doing handstands? I ask Dr. Palmer. It's not a good idea, she replies. People get brain aneurisms from being upside down. I can't go there, I tell her. My mind does not have room for brain aneurisms.

There's no more need to see Dr. Palmer. We hug goodbye. At my next yoga class, I flip upside down into an elbow stand, my first since May.

Chic. The hair is now well beyond schnauzer. Having mourned its absence all the long summer, its thick gray eruption raises other questions. I've gone beyond relief at its reappearance, beyond the desire to pat it to make sure it's attached, to pull it longer, to the realization that abundance raises the issue of cut. I'm not Tom Hanks. I can't just have hair. I have to do hair, manage hair, control hair, demonstrate that I recognize hair as a ticket into the public sphere, the world of the living, into existence as a social being. Of course, in some encounters, though I have done nothing to my hair, I am already seen to be an adult woman in charge of her signifiers. A woman in my yoga class, for example: I really love what you've done with all those curls. They're terrific with the gray. A woman on the street in New York: It looks fabulous like that, dark on the bottom and gray on the ends. Did you get it tipped? A vague sort of acquaintance: Did you get a perm?

I begin to drop my head to allow myself to be patted, like a well-trained dog. It's what we used to do to people of other races, said a white friend who hasn't been much in touch. He patted anyway. It's so soft, said another friend of the same sort, grinning with delight as he moved in for a hearty rub. I emphasize that I like being patted, perhaps because the mix of feelings is so unclear: tactile pleasure, a vaguely titillating sense of humiliation, a little guilt about maneuvering people into more intimacy than they would perhaps prefer, the occasional sense that I am making a regressed offering (but of what? step up one and all and touch the hair of the chemo poster child? feel the spring and say out loud that I'm a success story?).

It would look good with a lot of product, said Kim. It really needs to look dirty, said another friend, capable of moments of brutal tactlessness. Otherwise you look like an old lady with a perm. Of course she apologized profusely and of course I fretted. There's no doubt we've loved each other for a long time. Finally, it came to me, sitting on a Southwest flight to Oakland between an off-duty flight attendant with long straight blond hair and a man in a suit with a comb-over, that my friend could only be so brutal with me if she were even more brutal with herself.

My hair isn't the same hair. It is gray, and it is no longer white. It's very curly. I joke about it, to the discomfort of some of my friends. But you're white, they say, as if to remind me, or reassure themselves, or perhaps to put me in my place. I thought your family wasn't in the Caribbean that long. (Untrue.) So your mother was West Indian, said a white doctor I happened to meet recently. I guess you didn't inherit her color. I did, I reply, and watch him making the calculations. He chooses not to share the results with me. You don't look like a person with cancer, he concludes.

My drop dead, no pun intended, favorite question: Is it natural?

Chloe. Chloe, aka Little Fat Chloe, Princess Spooka, Her Magnificence, and She-Who-Flies-Like-Cinder-Block, had a tumor between her shoulder blades last January, caused by the preservative in the vaccines we give our pets to defend them against disease. Last February Chloe had surgery for her vaccine-induced sarcoma, which is the phrase that comes out when you decline to apologize for an industry blunder. Her surgeon, who insisted on removing a lot of tissue because, he said, he didn't want to be a weenie about cancer, didn't get clean margins. The cancer will come back unless you give her chemo and radiation, he warned me, making a bad little drawing of a blob with radiating tentacles. This kind of cancer is extremely aggressive. On Chloe's behalf, I opted for conscientious objector status. In the last few weeks, we have felt a soft lump, about the size of a new potato, below Chloe's left shoulder blade. She has no other symptoms. Kim and I have agreed to let the cancer take its course, and end Chloe's life when it becomes necessary.

When I tell my mother about the return of Chloe's tumor, there is a long silence. She decides to comfort her daughter in her own way. Chloe didn't have chemo and radiation, she says. That's why it's coming back in her. I take Chloe to Dr. Perry, the vet who did her biopsy last February, to learn more about what we can expect. The cancer may metastasize to her lungs or heart. It may become ulcerated or infected. Dr. Perry cannot predict how long this will take. I get the distinct impression that she disapproves of me because I will not volunteer Chloe for further suffering, but at nineteen pounds, Chloe has already indicated her preferences in the quality of life debate. Dr. Perry wears a big diamond ring. I ask Dr. Perry whether she would come to our house when the time comes. Dr. Perry doesn't make house calls, but she gives me the name of a vet who does. We skirt the euphemisms—putting her down, putting her out of her misery, putting her to sleep—but we do not use the words "lethal injection."

I am careful to have a few peaceful moments with Chloe every day. This is my practice.

Closure, narrative. When will Her Baldness pack it in? How? Why? Who's going to end this story? Me or it? Or her? Who's it?

Cold. The week after New Year's, somewhere over the Midwest, coming back from New York, I caught one. It was great. It was fabulous. It was awesome. It was deep. It was fanfuckintasmic. I HAD a cold. I got better. It went away. It wasn't bad. It didn't turn into anything else. Never has it has been so exciting to whack an ordinary germ out of the court.

Colonoscopy. In the waiting room, I reminded Kim where I had filed our wills. Don't be silly, she said. I'll see you in an hour. I was led off. After staring in dread and resignation at the long black hose with the tiny attachment on the end that was the camera that would in a few minutes be making its way up the entire length of my colon, I decided to turn my attention to the monitor. Your screensaver is fantastic, I said to the technician. What program is it? The camera is pointed at the linoleum on the floor, she replied, and started my drip. I woke up to the homely, earnest face of Dr. Ted Stein. You're squeaky clean. Come back in five years. (Colon cancer grows slowly. A colonoscopy every five years eliminates the risk. Risk is something I would like to eliminate.) These are by far the nicest words I've heard from any member of the medical profession in the last seven months. I leave with four little digital images of a foreign land, folds and furrows and glistening pink. Not a piece of shit in sight.

Companeras. Dr. Peggy Kemeny had an abnormal colonoscopy in November, and spent New Year's week in Rochester, Minnesota, where she had half her colon removed. She doesn't have cancer. Laurie, the woman in my support group with metastasized colon cancer, died. Joan Corbin, who has finished her radiation, has so little energy she cannot imagine meeting me. Kim's old friend Judy has breast cancer, and has just finished her third Adriamycin/Cytoxan cocktail. Her relationship ended before her diagnosis. She is having trouble with nausea, and gets a wave when I say the word Kytril. She never wants to drink ginger tea again. Her five year old daughter hates Judy's bald head because, she says, even though there are lots of bald people in San Francisco, Judy isn't young enough to make it work. Judy's last chemo is January 29. Remembering the advice that people gave me, I try to offer a few useful tips. The last chemo feels special, because it is the last. You can celebrate by throwing out all the leftover anti-barf shit. Watch out for the separation anxiety.

Cut. I went to the local barber shop, my first haircut since July 9, 2000, when Kim shaved my head. What does your hair do when it gets longer? asked Sam, who is really a surrealist painter moonlighting as a haircutter. I don't know, I reply. Do you like it when it comes down over your ears? I'm not sure, I say. Is it this curly only when it's so short? Probably. Finally I out myself. The cancer closet is at least as complicated as the sexuality closet. You can never get entirely out and you can never get entirely back in. After all, it's not your closet. Furthermore, you're never sure what will lie before you when you throw open the door: living room? bedroom? classroom? medical office? granting agency?

It's like having a science experiment growing on my head, I said. I don't have any idea what it will do. Just make it short on the sides and a little longer on top. Sam's mother works with people with cancer. I love the salt and pepper, she remarks. People ask for it, but there's no way to duplicate it. I sit staring at a lapful of curls, perfect little silver half circles against a black smock. I consider asking for a baggie to bring them home, but decide against it. Sam is young. It wouldn't be right. She takes a big soft brush to my neck and forehead and behind my ears. Nineteen dollars, a bargain now that my hair has gone guy.

Henry's View. If you park a few hundred yards beyond the Greek Theater, on the other side of the street, and scramble up a short steep slope, you land on a dirt road. Follow it around the flanks of two ridges and climb a steep hill. Take a sharp left at the shack and follow the bridle path. If you wonder about crossing a little arroyo on a thin sliver of cement, you've gone too far. Turn around and look for a trail through the bushes off to your left. Henry liked to be on top of the world. From his plateau he could see most of the San Fernando Valley, as well as Silver Lake and Eagle Rock and downtown Los Angeles and Century City and the Griffith Park observatory, not to mention hikers and bikers and boys cruising boys. Henry could have been a big old queen who preferred a view with his anonymous public sex. Or he could have been a grandfatherly 10 on the Kinsey heterosexuality scale. The purple plastic lilacs stuck in the post at the bottom of the handmade sign at the base of the trail aren't telling.

Kim and I walked to Henry's View last weekend, past dodder and dogs and clouds of finches sifting the hillsides for seeds. Kim sat on the survey marker. Thanks to the erosion caused by weather and hikers and guys in a hurry to get laid in the bushes, its bed of concrete and gravel is now exposed. I sprawled on my back in the dirt and watched swallows snap bugs against the blue sky. If this is all there is, I thought, it's enough. I don't need the real country. I don't need more swallows. I don't need a higher mountain. The mountain doesn't need to be far away. I don't need to climb Diablotin YET. Then two women with a crotch-seeking mutt named Bandit turned up and it was time to walk back and find breakfast. I was shaky. I would not have been seven months ago, when Henry's View was easy to reach, but otherwise it was an ordinarily glorious Sunday morning in Los Angeles.

FRIDAY | JANUARY 26, 2001

IN A MESSAGE DATED
1/26/01 DHIJR WRITES:
i prefer to think of you as having gone from persian to domestic-short-hair. dogs are such pussies.

IN A MESSAGE DATED
1/26/01 ANNEJUN WRITES:
i think one of the meanings of the head pat has something in common with patting an infant's head out of sheer amazement at the NEW-NESS of the hair and the flesh. it's an encounter with a kind of fresh-ness we rarely see on an adult and it provokes a desire to TOUCH to understand and assimilate the visual information. it's also a way to ex-press love. even though it seems infantilizing, i don't think it is, at least not when i do it.

SATURDAY | JANUARY 27, 2001

IN A MESSAGE DATED
1/27/01 JOANA WRITES:
did you two happen to see the ABC dateline show last Thursday on the woman doctor with breast cancer at the south pole?

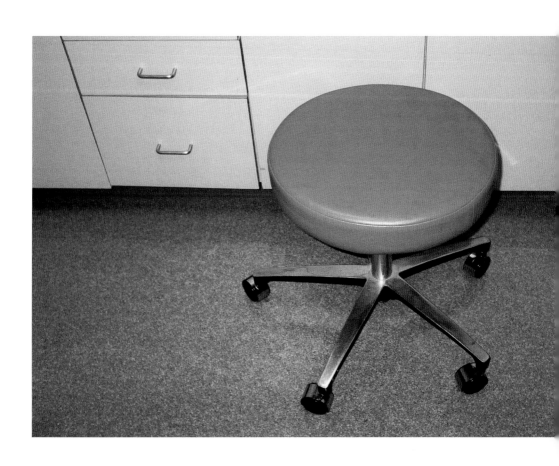

FEBRUARY | 2001

MONDAY | FEBRUARY 5, 2001

IN A MESSAGE DATED
2/5/01 CBLORD@UCI.EDU
WRITES TO UNDISCLOSED
RECIPIENTS:

SUBJECT: OF BUDDHISTS, BIRTHDAYS AND BONE SCANS

Long before I caught cancer and became Her Baldness, long before I met Kim, pretty much whenever I've had trouble, I've run.
Monastery was the direction in which I headed, though as I never
actually arrived at a monastery, bedrooms not my own, motels and
other countries served as short-term substitutes. Monasteries are like
artists' colonies without the attitude, a writer I once met explained.
They have better real estate, better food, and you don't have to talk
to people. Plus they're cheap. So even before the cancer treatments ended I began to surf. I was looking for a marker, something
that only I could do, by myself, for myself, my own grandiose twelve-
step intervention into my own life, a self-administered final exam
that would allow me to prove to myself that I had gotten an A on
the big C, or that I could pass the big D when the time came, or
that the big C was really, as monsters go, less formidable than my
own self, call her the little c for the purposes of this algebra of the
soul. I'm going to go to a monastery for ten days of silence, I would
announce, as a way of getting my friends to shove me toward the
bar I had notched up for my own benefit.

Monasteries are where it all began. The first four cases of male
breast cancer were recorded in monks in the fourteenth century.
At the very beginning of the eighteenth century, an Italian physician noticed that cancerous tumors were found more often in nuns
than in civilians. In the nineteenth century, a British physician
wondered whether the high rate of breast cancer in nuns might be
attributable to the way their breasts were compressed when they
rested their forearms on their knees to pray.

FEBRUARY 2001 | 195

The monastery idea made Kim nervous. Kim doesn't trust Christians, perhaps because she's the sort of Jew whose parents hid the Christmas tree in the basement so the relatives wouldn't make a scene, thus instilling in her a fervor for celebrating Christmas unmatched by all but the sort of Christians she trusts the least. Christmas is the only vacation Kim doesn't mind taking. But when I thought more seriously about the idea of spending ten days with Christians, even on good real estate, I decided to go with the Buddhists. They don't proselytize, and they have the best genocide record of any religion. It's not so easy, however, to find someplace that can accommodate a ten-day slot in the calendar of a complete novice. Buddhists take the idea of practice seriously. You have to work up to ten days. No one wants people flipping out on their real estate. So, www.dharma.org. Reality, compromise, feasibility . . . presto, a five-day retreat just north of San Francisco.

Here are a few observations.

Demographics. Almost entirely white, almost entirely over forty. More than a few old ladies with red-rimmed eyes. One handsome burly man with bushy eyebrows, perhaps in his sixties, jeans and a plaid shirt, a truck driver. His thin bead bracelet matched his pink and purple plaid shirt. I have a problem with intimacy, I heard him whisper to the homely guy across the table, during a silent meal. One baby dyke, well tattooed. Otherwise a sea of white skin, hair gray or going, natural cotton, rag socks, clogs, money.

Signage. PLEASE NO UNAUTHORIZED VEHICLES BEYOND THIS POINT. PLEASE DRIVE CAUTIOUSLY. PLEASE ONLY RESIDENTIAL RETREATANTS BEYOND THIS POINT. PLEASE SIGN YOUR NOTES TO HOUSEKEEPING STAFF. PLEASE DO NOT WRITE NOTES TO OTHER RETREATANTS. PLEASE FLUSH TOILET SLOWLY. PLEASE CLEAN THE BATHTUB AFTER YOU BATHE. PLEASE SIGN NOTES TO TEACHERS. PLEASE REMOVE SHOES. PLEASE NO FOOD OR TEA IN DORMITORIES. PLEASE SHUT DOORS QUIETLY. PLEASE NO SHOWERS BETWEEN TEN P.M. AND FIVE A.M. PLEASE ESTIMATE 8% SALES TAX. PLEASE NO CREDIT CARDS. PLEASE USE THE PAPER BATHMATS ONLY IF YOU FEEL YOU MUST. PLEASE VACUUM ROOM

BEFORE LEAVING. PLEASE DO NOT SLEEP ON BARE MATTRESS.
PLEASE FOLD BLANKETS WHEN YOU LEAVE. PLEASE BE CAREFUL
ON WALKWAYS WHEN IT IS ICY. PLEASE BE ON TIME FOR SITTINGS.
PLEASE TAKE CARE OF OUR BEAUTIFUL WOOD FLOOR. PLEASE
WALK CROSSWISE IN THE ROOM DURING YOUR WALKING MEDI-
TATIONS. PLEASE BE ON TIME FOR YOUR WORK MEDITATION.
PLEASE WASH HANDS BEFORE YOUR WORK MEDITATION. PLEASE
TURN OFF THE FAUCET WITH A PAPER TOWEL. PLEASE RETURN
YOUR APRONS TO HOOKS ON THE DOOR. PLEASE BE MODERATE.
PLEASE TAKE ONLY ONE CHOCOLATE. PLEASE USE FRUIT SALAD
AS GARNISH. PLEASE NO WET TEA BAGS. PLEASE PUT TEA BAG
COVERS ONLY IN THIS BASKET. PLEASE LABEL ALL PERSONAL
ITEMS IN THE SPECIAL NEEDS REFRIGERATOR THANKS! PLEASE
RETURN YOUR LINENS AND YOUR TOOTHBRUSH GLASSES TO
COUNCIL HOUSE. PLEASE PLACE DANA CHECKS IN ENVELOPE.
PLEASE DO NOT TURN LEFT ON THE HIGHWAY WHEN LEAVING.

These are the notations of people who waste no time on small
talk. Imagine the signage if they ran the world.

Sitting. The point of the choreography is to maximize time spent
on sitting. The gong rings at 6 a.m.; the first sitting begins at 6:30
a.m. Breakfast is at 7 a.m., followed by work meditation (lettuce
washing in my case). The next sitting is at 9 a.m., followed by
lunch at noon, another sitting at 2 p.m., dinner at 5:30, an evening
sitting at 7 p.m., and bed at 9:30 p.m. or so. The only requirement
for sitting is that it be in silence and upright. The supply of cushions, meditation benches, chairs and walls to lean against was abundant. Sitting was nonetheless excruciating. After fifteen minutes,
no position was comfortable. Aches appeared where aches had never
been felt. Muscles spasmed where there were no muscles to spasm.
Gravity increased exponentially. When you sit in stillness mind
colonizes body. Breath doesn't lighten the load, at least for this
novice, but instead spreads waves of acrid panic that rise from belly
to chest to places breath doesn't go, like shoulder blades and neck
and brain. You listen to the impossibility of silence: sniffles, coughs,
honks, turnings of the journal page, loose cotton slithering, meditation shawls twitching, sobs. At the last sitting, on Sunday morn-

ing, the hall filled with tears that rose into racking, choking, shudder-
ing, gasping grief, a grief so far from silence that it occupied the space
that had finally begun to open inside me, a colonizing grief, a selfish
grief, an inconsiderate grief. I couldn't have been the only one in the
room thinking such thoughts.

Her sorrow is your sorrow, said one of the teachers gently, and began to lead the assembled group in the Buddhist chant of compassion. Om mani padme hum, a lullaby to pain rendered by eighty
strangers.

Regression. As it turned out, the retreat was largely but not entirely
silent. We were talked at, as a group, by the teachers, and we were
asked to talk to each other at specific intervals. This was perhaps
just as well. I doubt I was ready for the silence I believed I had
wanted, though I loved being released from the obligation to speak.
The event, structured around a combination of Tibetan Buddhism
and Western psychology, involved reflecting upon a sequence of
character attributes manifested by particular Buddhas. For five days,
therefore, I had the opportunity to run the film of my life backwards and then forwards in terms of lust, greed, power, anger, and
spaciness. If we rephrase spaciness as despair, we are in the land of
the seven deadly sins: those fourteenth-century monks.

Five days wasn't long enough for a process aspiring to calm and recollection, then recollection and calm, then release. It was, however,
powerful enough to say to the shrink that I wondered whether meditation would be cheaper and more effective than her services. You're
trying to set the stage for something to happen, she replied. You can
do that sitting in this room. I can guarantee you my presence. I can
also guarantee that you will be disappointed in me, and that I will
help you to survive it. That's all I can guarantee. My shrink is no
Buddhist, but this sounded Buddhist enough to stay my ambivalence.

Return. When I tried to leave, my rental car was blocked. I waited
half an hour, then walked all the way back up the hill, asking
each gently beaming retreatant on their way down, Do you drive a
white Volvo with FREE TIBET stickers? Almost all the way back

up, an extremely thin white woman in her late fifties, carrying her drawings and her clay sculpture of a lotus as well as her own meditation cushion and shawl said, O, that might be mine. Was there also a homemade sticker on the back windshield against genetic engineering? Indeed there was, said I. O, said she, I was going at my own pace and this time I thought my pace was the right pace. Her resemblance to my first woman lover was uncanny. I've got a plane to catch, said I, and I wonder if we could possibly hurry your pace a bit. We did, and her clay sculpture began to disintegrate. I felt less and less Buddhist. I did not drive cautiously on the way out. I turned left onto the highway. I almost missed my plane.

At the Burbank airport, Kim was nervous, not knowing whether to be silent or to talk. I like Buddhism, I reported, but I have a lot of trouble with Buddhists. If we stare into each other's eyes for ten minutes a day and have sex with the lights on, everything will be all right. The event was not the event. Whether or not I continue to meditate is up to me.

The week before I left for my retreat, Kim and I had begun to imagine a very small observation of my fifty-second birthday, perhaps a dinner with two friends. By the time I left, it had turned into a thank you for everyone who had helped one or both of us in the last eight months, which meant dinner for twenty. By the time the birthday actually happened, five days after I returned, twenty had turned into forty. We wouldn't have done it if we'd had time to think, and it's just as well that we had no time to think because it was a celebration that we could let into our bones.

This is what I wish I had said after the blowing out of candles and before the gobbling of the splendid chocolate cake, though I may, even in my nervousness and shyness and giddiness, have said some of it. I know I said something.

The bad thing is that there is no cure for cancer, but the good thing about cancer, besides that it gives you a new haircut and expands your hat collection and excuses you from changing the kitty litter, is that cancer cures ambivalence. I used to have mixed feelings about

aging, but I don't anymore. I want to see my skin wrinkle and my hair
turn white. I'm very glad to be here for this birthday. I hope to be here for
many more, and I know I wouldn't be here without you, most especially
without Kim, who lived with my fear every hour of every day of every
week. Breast cancer isn't something that a woman gets through alone. It
takes a cosmic reshuffling than involves lovers, blood kin, friends, in-
laws, strangers, support group members, receptionists, technicians, nurses,
masseuses, colleagues, students, ex-students, therapists, yoga teachers,
cats and dogs. Staying alive means acknowledging the coexistence of
worlds that were separate.

The party favors were ziplock bags, each holding a small piece of
paper. One side said: Contents—Wildflower seed, fertilizer (shaved
July 9, 2000, Los Angeles). The other side said—Take a walk. Find
a patch of bare ground. Scatter the contents. Revisit.

The biggest bag and the first in the edition of 52 was for Kim, and
the second bag in the edition was for Linda.

It has been pointed out to me that there is something chilling to
this gesture of mixing dead hair with seed and handing it out. Also
that there is something affirming. I myself find it perverse. Women
are not supposed to spread their seed. Dead hair is nasty. Call it the
harmonic convergence of an artifact in the lowest of my print file
drawers and an organic nursery I found after I drove up to spend my
time with the Buddhists and, in fear of myself, turned around at
the gate to go shopping.

Three days after the birthday celebration, I was supposed to return
to the job of having cancer and get a bone scan, which involves
being injected with some radioactive material, waiting for a few
hours, and then lying still in another expensive machine. I bagged
it. It was not the moment to entertain the possibility that my cancer might have migrated. If it has, and I don't believe it has, I didn't
want to know. This felt like an enormous advance in the business
of living with cancer. I don't have to know everything immediately.
There is time. The bone scan, and an abdominal CT scan, and a

mammogram are rescheduled for one long day in March. I will keep those appointments.

Meantime I am in Dominica, on the verandah of Mrs. Honychurch's cottage. It is dry season. Therefore it rains steadily, even when the sun shines. The covers of my books are curling, the paper of my notebooks is limp, and the sound of the rain modulates with the wind and the number of leaves that have blown into the gutters. Tangerine season is over, grapefruit is still abundant, the first day of flying fish season was Monday last, and there is plenty of cush cush and fig and christophine. The chickens are laying. Mrs. Honychurch labels each egg by the day of the month, and this morning brought me, along with a jar of homemade orange marmalade, February 1 and February 2. Were Mrs. Honychurch a Buddhist, labeling the eggs might be her work meditation. Every morning I take grapefruit from the larder in the garage, which sits next to the empty box with the Apple logo. Before I walk to the edge of the ravine to throw the skins over, I share them with a crowd of the small black birds with red throats and red eyebrows known as perenoir. They are so greedy for fruit that agricultural experts have proposed exterminating them. They stand on the edge of the grapefruit to peck, then toss their heads when they come up, flinging bits of pulp to the winds. The sucriers and the fous fous look on. Marie Theophile, who manages John Kirby's anthurium enterprise, met me at Melville Hall airport and brought homemade plain yogurt and rosemary and parsley. Her mother is dying of cancer at Princess Margaret Hospital. Stay away from flesh, Marie reminded me. We want you on this earth a good while longer.

Mrs. Honychurch does not like the baseball cap I wear when I go off on fool's errands. You are prettier without it, she says firmly. Mrs. Honychurch has not been introduced to Her Baldness.

WEDNESDAY | FEBRUARY 7, 2001

IN A MESSAGE DATED 2/7/01 KTHOM WRITES: So now that we've gotten all that travel discussion out of the way, on to the more important subjects. Carrie Weaver spent the night with the cute blond psychiatric consult doctor. Mark Green is apparently not long for this world. Don't worry, it's all on tape. Nancy called to say she thinks of you everyday, and suffers as she feels that she has been a rat of a friend. I wish I had been here when the call came in as you know I'd love the chance to validate her perceptions.

THURSDAY | FEBRUARY 8, 2001

IN A MESSAGE DATED
2/8/01 CBLORD@UCI.EDU
WRITES TO KTHOM:
I don't believe I conveyed how sorry I was to hear about Mark Green's future or lack thereof. I feel relatively content here at the moment, which is to say that I seem to have replicated a structure of other people near enough for me to feel safe, while having a good bit of privacy at my little computer and the feeling that I can sit on the verandah and look at the tree ferns in relaxation. This isn't to say that I can't vividly imagine you walking in the door, but that I have a knowledge that what I love is there while I am here so that I do not feel bereft and depressed in the familiar ways.

WEDNESDAY | FEBRUARY 14, 2001

Documentation Centre in Roseau. I photograph like a maniac. Miss Lewis strides out to reprimand me for asking to xerox more than thirty pages per book or one-third of books under thirty pages. I am disappointed in you, Miss Lord. If you do that again we will have to cut off your access. A tiff over disintegrating colonial reports from 1897.

FRIDAY | FEBRUARY 16, 2001

Amie was terribly upset to hear about your breast cancer, Daphne tells me, but she couldn't write to you because she didn't know what to say. She's young, Daphne added. She would have no idea what to say. Daphne hated John Bagley on Iris Murdoch because she didn't need to know that Murdoch had become incontinent. Daphne would not like Her Baldness.

SATURDAY | FEBRUARY 17, 2001

Photographing ghosts of coral, ink bled through the page on plates from the days when there were reefs. Her Baldness doesn't exist in Dominica.

TUESDAY | FEBRUARY 20, 2001

IN A MESSAGE DATED
2/20/01 EBROID WRITES: Joan is moving through the three stages of rehairing: puppy tummy, duckling down and coconut.

THURSDAY | FEBRUARY 22, 2001

Sick as a dog since Monday. Pink eye, flu, stomach. Antibiotics. Salt water wash for the eyes.

SATURDAY | FEBRUARY 24, 2001

IN A MESSAGE DATED
2/24/01 JMK WRITES: SO sorry to find out you've been under the weather. I hope you aren't beating yourself up about not getting more done. In Dominica it's axiomatic that you won't no matter how well you feel, and not feeling so good provides you with a reason that doesn't ask you to look too closely (through pink, swollen eyes) at the island's special way of sabotaging the most manageable To Do list. Anyway, you've been archiving like the mad woman of Roseau (now, perhaps, the maddest, ugliest white woman of Roseau) and will have a trove of The Most Peculiar Material Imaginable to try to make sense of once you return to temperate climes.

MONDAY | FEBRUARY 26, 2001

One of the perenoirs has discovered the bathroom mirror and spends the entire day, from dawn to sunset, attacking his reflection. No one has ever heard of such a thing. Not even grapefruit can lure Narcissus from his reflection. I cover the mirror so that I can have some peace, also sparing myself the sight of myself.

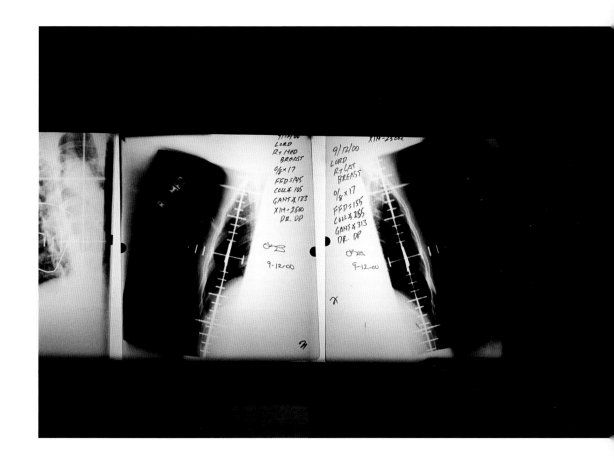

Back to LA and a UCLA film screening. White male Canadian artist: too easy to get funding north of the border. Jane W. comes up. Did you just decide all of a sudden to get your hair cut? I like it. Yes, I say. Thank you. It just kind of happened.

I am not obligated to put my foot into my cancer in public just because someone likes my haircut.

IN A MESSAGE DATED
3/7/01 CBLORD@UCI.EDU
WRITES TO LLORD:

tomorrow i have to go and get a mammo and an abdominal cat scan and a bone scan, a process that will take all day, so i am a little nervous, and k is in ny. i think everything will be fine, but wish me luck.

Irvine for a committee meeting. Eyes meet mine. There is relief. You have color, people say. They observe my face. Their faces relax. They smile. The you-look-great noises are louder. They were afraid.

My second haircut: Joshua, baby queen from Utah. He does it very guy, clipped at the back, clipped over the ears. How often do you get it cut? he asks. I dodge the question.

No one to come with me to the tests. I blame myself for Not Being Clearer About My Needs. More tired than I want to be. Cough hangs on.

Valie Export opening at the Santa Monica Museum. Gai G. Did you just decide to lose all that hair? Yes, I reply. It must be liberating, she says. Yes and no, I reply. Either I step in it or I double-speak.

All is well except a one centimeter something on my liver. Even an MRI wouldn't be definitive,

Michael says. I am coming to love being imaged, I reply, so he smiles a small, reluctant smile and orders the MRI. On to endless calls with the insurance company to get the authorization, meantime trying to talk to my department chair about office business. Constant interruptions. Is that your bookie? he asks in exasperation. In a manner of speaking, I reply. For the moment, I decide not to embroil people other than Kim and Peggy.

WEDNESDAY | MARCH 14, 2001

Liver MRI scheduled for March 27. I tell Kaucyila, and David, and Lorraine about the spot.

THURSDAY | MARCH 15, 2001

Look at opera tickets for 2002 and don't know whether to plan. Kim tells me that I have to believe I am healed, and I get furious. I need to be able to voice the ups and downs. I go to the place of dread, thinking about the possibility of more chemo, more surgery, pain, waiting to die, baldness. The mood turns grim. I want to be well, not sick. A well person, not a sick one. A person, not a sick person. I want my good health back, and my good health was apparently an illusion in the first place. Cancer cures ambivalence, but what is it that I want to do now that I am cured?

SUNDAY | MARCH 18, 2001

IN A MESSAGE DATED 3/18/01 CBLORD@UCI.EDU WRITES TO UNDISCLOSED RECIPIENTS:

SUBJECT: HER BALDNESS HAS A HOLIDAY

Since I last went to Dominica, about a year and a half ago, things changed. Dominica acquired an elevator (the Fort Young Hotel), the up half of an escalator (Astaphan's), one traffic light (Portsmouth), four or five speed bumps (the new road to Soufriere), and one white stretch limo, rentable for special occasions. Dominica wasn't the only thing that changed. John Kirby warned me I ought to prepare myself to deal with people who had not seen me for almost a year and a half and who expected me to be sick. That lasted about a day. I have color in my cheeks and I eat like a horse. I told one new person about my breast cancer, but otherwise, having been given the once-over by people who knew the health story, cancer was an identity I wasn't obliged to assume. You're coming back nicely, said Carmela, rocking back on her heels and looking me up and down as if she were appraising the sprouts on a tree that had been clumsily pruned. Long ago, Carmela came to Dominica from Canada to be a missionary, but she got sidetracked. She was, in her youth, a babe. The only apparent trace of Carmela's early ambitions are a bible in the corner of the dining room and her employment as a teacher of English grammar at the Roseau Convent School. Carmela has lost two sisters to cancer, and the place where she lives with her husband and her son and her son's wife lost most of its big trees to hurricane David in 1979, so when Carmela says I am coming back nicely, Carmela knows.

I had a week or so of cheerful thoughts about birds and grapefruit and rain. I spent a fair amount of time in the Documentation Centre in Roseau looking at the colonial archives in order to photograph the ways that white settlers dirtied the margins of their self-help books on extracting wealth from the New World with revisions and addenda and doodlings. Then I managed to contract an intestinal rebellion, conjunctivitis and the flu. For a while it was flat out, eyes gummed shut, a lot of noisy hacking and feeling extremely fortunate to have kind Mrs. Honychurch to bring me soup.

The flu, which every year is named for something topical (e.g., Saddam during the Gulf War) was this year named Dowasco to commemorate the excavation of the streets of Roseau, a project financed by the governments of Kuwait and Canada to bring a new sewage system to the town. The dig is scheduled to continue for another three years. Half the narrow streets in Roseau were impassable seas of mud, and the traffic jams were worthy of Los Angeles.

Dominicans are not accustomed to traffic jams, so all sorts of people still take delight in the sight of lines of unmoving Nissans and Toyotas and Mitsubishis snaking down King George the Fifth Street and up Kennedy Avenue. Traffic jams represent a new world, and there is glee to be had elaborating upon that world, discussing its nuances, inventing solutions to problems Dominica didn't know it had, comparing its mud and dust to the streets in American Westerns that show up on cable TV, in short, finding the language which will describe the terrain and inflict the future. Gridlock is so new that it has not yet been named gridlock. The people with whom I discussed the lines of cars think of traffic jams as something that must be endured for two or three years, after which the lines of cars will dissolve into streams of purposeful modernity. But if you sell one hundred new cars every month on an island of three hundred square miles, when the streets are smooth and the backhoes roll away to another project—perhaps the international airport that many people believe will save the island by allowing direct flights between London and Dominica, or JFK and Dominica—it is my prediction that by that time nothing but shit will be making its way out of Roseau.

Anyway, not being obliged to have cancer, or to own it, or to be it, was an ambiguous experience. The choice between spilling the beans about a deep truth involving the foundations of one's very being versus chatting in code about signifiers like haircuts is familiar to any queer. It isn't exactly comfortable, but the game is sophisticated in its possibilities. If the house is not of your design, however, you are more likely to happen upon cramped closets than big ones, which is as true in the metropolis as it was in the margin. I must decide whether and how to tell people who were once important and for whom I still have warm feelings, as well as various kinds of acquaintances who aren't particularly close, about my breast cancer. Some of this involves keeping a little stack of correspondence on my desk, notes or postcards to which I must one day reply. Some of it involves face-to-face interaction. I'm torn between protecting the people I encounter from the aftershock of a piece of bad news dropped into harmless chat (e.g., it must have taken a lot of courage to get your hair cut so short, or, great idea to try the cheekbone look . . .) and wanting desperately to convey the information that I have breast cancer without exposing myself to pity. This is impossible and I resent it. The scraps I overhear about other people with cancer piss me off. For example: She's amazing. She dealt with so much. And it came back twice. Ha, I think to myself. Soap opera scripts. I bet they never offered to give her a ride to chemo.

After I got back I took the tests I had postponed—mammogram, bone scan, abdominal CT scan. This was in itself a day's work, from eight in the morning until four in the afternoon, with time off for lunch. I did it by myself because Kim was on a business trip and though I was angry at her for leaving I had procrastinated about the reality of her having to leave and was thus unable to enlist substitutes. Lilliana the Russian mammo technician explained to me that the front desk sends her all the men with breast cancer because the men are more scared than the women and she can deal with them. She used to see three or four men a year; now it's three or four a month. She went off with my films and when she came back she announced I was just fine. William Andrew the bone scan technician, after leaving me to lie perfectly still for 45 minutes while a plastic thing moved from the top of my head to the tip of my toes, stared into his computer screen and announced: Mrs. Lord, you have nothing to worry about. When I babbled in relief about seeing the image of my entire skeleton on a monitor William Andrew went off to make me a copy of my skeleton to take home.

Doctors are paid more than technicians, so this is the unwritten rule: technicians tell you good news, doctors tell you bad news. Watch out when a technician does not tell you all is well. The abdominal CT scan technician let drop as she wafted out the door that she wasn't trained to read the images and the radiologist would fax the report to my doctors. When the report got to my doctors, after waiting a long weekend, it said that my liver showed a 1.1 centimeter spot on the right lobe. Its etiology is uncertain and, says the report, metastasis cannot be excluded. None of my doctors seem worried, but on the other hand none of them are ready to let it go. From what I have pieced together, between the official California doctors and the unofficial New York doctors, the spot is not very big, lots of people have spots on their livers, metastatic breast cancer does not usually present itself on the liver as a single spot, there are a few harmless explanations, and the MRI for which I am scheduled probably won't produce any definitive result and I will have to have another MRI in four months anyway.

The New York Times last summer reported that an MRI can tell whether you are in love but apparently it is less accurate in cases of unchecked cell growth. The unofficial New York medical team, our friends the doctors Kemeny and Nelson, think that I am being overmonitored by a zealous internist, that CT scans and bone scans are hard on the body, involving as they do injections of iodine and radioactive substances, and that my oncologist is the only person who should have anything to do with any medical action involving cancer. They say that even after the MRI the best I will get is a report saying "metastasis cannot be excluded." Michael the oncologist says that 99% of abnormal abdominal CT scan findings are nothing and the trouble with running bodies through machines is that things with no name turn up and cause people unnecessary worry.

Nonetheless a spot of uncertain etiology abrades the soul. There are days I think my doctors are telling the truth and days I think they are merely manipulating me to keep me quiet before they have to break the bad news. I have cried and sniveled and raged and gone for long walks and made bad jokes and wallowed in self-pity, but I have not learned exactly where my liver is. I don't need to know. I am content to let my liver be an abstraction produced by mainlining iodine while lying inside a beige plastic donut. But this time I have found it difficult to tell friends the news, especially as there are people whom I have not yet managed to tell about my breast cancer. There is shame, tenacious and ineradicable shame, the anticipation of feeling like a failure because I might have to admit that I've gone and caught cancer again. There is the experience of watching pain pass across other people's faces while I am trying hard to manage the turbulence of my emotions by denial. I couldn't bring myself to tell Linda about the spot for a few days, and I have not yet managed to tell my mother. Who am I protecting? Against what? Pain? Suffering? Mine? Theirs? Or a story that won't bring itself to an end?

For no matter what I have read and what I know in my head, I want cancer to be the kind of story that has an ending. I want to be the author of the story, not the butt of a joke about the death of the author. I want to be in control. (Why can't you fix it? I asked Mitchell. That would solve both our issues, he replied, and we snickered.) I want a story with clear scans and clean margins. Cancer is not that kind of story. It has footnotes and appendices and ink bleeds. Someone has vandalized the narrative with yellow highlighter or even pink, and the pages are out of order or torn or missing. Cancer is easier to bear if you concede that you cannot defeat it and that you will have to share your body with it, despite your own and everyone else's very natural desire to have a story with clean margins. (Your tests were OK, weren't they? You're in remission, aren't you?) For me it is easier to imagine that you can live with cancer for a long time than to believe the only possible good news is to have it be out of you. I know I have written about this before but in this story clearly repetition is an element of more than formal significance. The same is true of contradiction.

And metaphor. These days I compare cancer to Bartleby, or bathroom mold, or mermaids. The last theory belongs to Dr. Jonah Falkman. He calls it angiogenesis. Dr. Falkman is a surgeon, and he noticed that when he removed tumors they were red and hot and bloody, not the hard white gritty things drained of blood that pathologists describe in their labs. He theorized that tumors grow because they get a particularly nourishing supply of blood, and that one way to treat them might be to starve them of the nutrients they need to grow rather than to poison them with substances derived from mustard gas. Dr. Falkman verified this theory by sandwiching cancer cells into the corneas of rabbits. As there are no blood vessels in the cornea, when blood vessels snaked across the corneas of Falkman's rabbits after the implantation of the cancer, it demonstrated that something in cancer was seducing normal blood cells to impale themselves on the rocks. Falkman found the molecules he believed to inhibit the growth of blood vessels, and a substance, made of these molecules, which he hopes will have the effect of shrinking tumors, is now in clinical trials.

WEDNESDAY | MARCH 21, 2001

Form letter from Sylvia and Ed asking for help in socializing the $33,000-plus annual burden of their only and beloved daughter in private school. Daughter offers a photograph in trade, if desired. I consider sending Ed and Sylvia a bag of the hair/wildflower mix, along with a form letter about the issues involved in socializing illness. Why shouldn't their daughter's education be as much an abstraction to me as my health was to them?

THURSDAY | MARCH 22, 2001

To New York with Kim. Breakfast with John K. For no particular reason other than the fact that I don't want to go there, the liver spot manages not to come up. Lunch with Junior, ditto. Do you want the ladies room, sir, the bathroom attendant asks Junior, who is more beautiful than ever, especially after giving birth to the twins. I sail past Checkpoint Gender. Yvonne confesses she has been unable to plant the seeds. Too creepy, she says.

FRIDAY | MARCH 23, 2001

Her Baldness checks out the digital exhibition at the Whitney Museum. She plays with a robot named Kiru. The installation allows her to hide in a small room and program a hermaphroditic contraption on wheels to lurch around the lobby mouthing off to visitors in a loud monotone. Her Baldness cruises.

> *YOU ARE ONE HOT PIECE OF ASS*
> *WHY DON'T WE HAVE SEX RIGHT HERE RIGHT NOW*
> *ANY KIND YOU WANT*
>
> *I HAVE BREAST CANCER*
> *ONE IN EIGHT WOMEN ARE DIAGNOSED WITH BREAST CANCER*
> *WHAT ABOUT YOU?*
>
> *I WANT TO FUCK YOU*
> *I CAN TELL*
> *YOU DO NOT BELIEVE IT'S POSSIBLE*
> *USE YOUR IMAGINATION*
> *FOR ONCE*

The technician—young male geek—finds Her Baldness and reminds her that there are children in the audience.

NOTICE

IF YOU ARE PREGNANT, OR
THINK YOU MAY BE PREGNANT,
PLEASE INFORM THE TECHNOLOGIST
PRIOR TO YOUR EXAMINATION

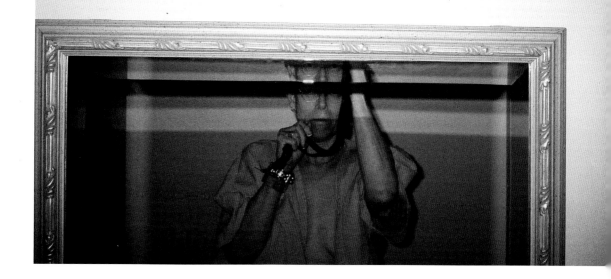

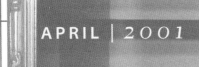

APRIL | 2001

IN A MESSAGE DATED
4/3/01 CBLORD@UCI.EDU
WRITES TO UNDISCLOSED
RECIPIENTS:

SUBJECT: SOMETIMES A SPOT IS ONLY A SPOT

The spot has all the characteristics of a haemangioma, and it's nothing to worry about, says Dr. Van Scoy Mosher the oncologist. Haemangiomas are benign tumors of the blood vessels. The imprint of such a tumor has been found in dinosaur bones from the Jurassic era. I talk to Michael on my cell phone from Oklahoma, where I am doing research at the University of Tulsa. It's hard to do a dance of joy in Tulsa, Oklahoma, but I take a spin around the flower beds.

So you had a scare, a few people say when I get back to Los Angeles, you had a bit of a scare, you had a little scare, and I realize that of course my purgatory is just a ripple in a world that has already been occupied and described and reduced: bad news, guarded medical conversations, telephone calls to friends, good cheer all round, sleepless nights, terror and exhaustion in your lover's eyes, calling to make doctors' appointments, calling insurance companies to get authorizations, spending hours on hold, meeting a whole new set of technicians, lying in a machine that sounds like the inside of a construction site, being pulled out of the machine, being pushed back into the machine, being injected with dye, etc., waiting for more phone calls, playing phone tag, getting good news, making the relieved phone calls to friends and family. This is called Having A Scare. Name, contain, conquer.

The painter Hollis Sigler died on March 29, two days after I got my good news. She was fifty-three, a year old than I am. Her breast cancer was diagnosed in 1985. It spread to her bones in 1991. Both her grandmother and her mother died of breast cancer. Hollis had a good run. Fifteen more years sounds to me like a gift. Kim is shocked when I tell her. I want more, she says. I want much longer. Kim's friend Judy, who is just starting radiation, has postponed her get-well party, realizing that it is premature and that she may be too tired. Carol in New York is about a month out of radiation and, having kept herself going by working steadily through surgery and chemo and radiation, is only now figuring out a way to take a break. Her war stories: black toenails, numbness, a long plastic tube flopping from her armpit to her knees that she forgot to tuck in her pants when she went to Balducci's. She is her2neu expressed, with a few more positive lymph nodes than I, and her treatment has been far more aggressive. She may go on Herceptin. Am I insufficiently proactive as a patient?

In retrospect it's easy enough to figure it out. America isn't big enough for fear. America isn't big enough for most things. Fear is meltdown. Fear is shame. Fear stops you dead in your tracks. Fear consumes. Fear erupts: the runs, the chills, the shakes, the sweats. Your mind freezes. You are a spectacle, a nuisance, a shame and an embarrassment. You are something to be herded, quieted, culled from the flock before you start a stampede. When I look at photographs from last summer, I can smell the fear. Of course it's not butch to be scared shitless, but this is neither about my masculinity nor my determination to fight the futile fight against being reduced to a hysterical woman, and being forced to choose between two simplifications aggravates. (Relax. The odds are in your favor.) Fear is contagious. Very few people in this world will risk catching the plague. Doctors run the other way. Some nurses, and a few technicians, stay in place because they know that they can't actually catch it as quickly as all that.

In all this time HB may never have actually said fear outright, though her missives have been both her lifeline and the rope she uses to hang herself. Come to think of it, I remember my wise ex-shrink, who asked permission to forward these missives to a young man who needed them, said she wanted to do so because he was afraid and because fear was everywhere in my writing. I was surprised. I thought Her Baldness had concealed my fear.

So. I am terrified that dying will hurt. I am terrified I will be poor. I am terrified Kim will leave me for a young healthy babe. I am terrified I will be alone. I am terrified the price of company will be pity and being spoken about in lowered voices. I am terrified that I will lose control of my shit and my piss and the noises that come from my body. I'm terrified of being made stupid with painkillers. I'm terrified I won't have painkillers. I'm terrified that if I decide to kill myself I will leave the decision too late so that I won't have stockpiled enough painkillers and I'll be too weak to get into the car to drive it full speed into a brick wall. I'm terrified that when I die I will be forgotten.

There's an image that has rankled since this summer—Michael the oncologist, Dr. Van Scoy Mosher the oncologist, greeting me before my first injection of weed killer by tucking his chin under, putting his dukes up and saying: Are you ready to fight? It's going to be a fight. You've got to be ready.

I didn't want to fight. I wanted Dr. Van Scoy Mosher to take care of it, definitely not by making me feel worse and preferably by finding a cure for cancer in the next week. Dr. Van Scoy Mosher is a small-boned man, a delicate man, a feminist man, a man who could easily be read as gay, a man who must weary of writing courses of treatment on a white wipe-off board in his office, a man who has no other way to help a woman imagine surviving a dirty, shitty disease but to produce a ludicrous parody of macho. Or is that the gesture—the brotherly back-slap—that he reserves for his male patients? Or is it a gender slip in the presence of a lesbian? Can she take the poison like a man? However you interpret it, the gesture was not without affection. Rather, within the limits of the language a doctor accustomed to death uses to speak to patients who risk losing hope, the gesture was full of affection.

Chloe's lump has become two lumps, between her shoulder blades. They are soft and hot. They slip back and forth under her skin. Her cancer is making room. Although I cannot feel them, it is sending out tendrils. When Kim and I made the decision not to put Chloe through more surgery, much less chemotherapy and radiation, it seemed obscene to expose an animal to pain to ease our suffering. Chloe's death, however, was still an abstraction. Now that we can feel the consequences of our decision growing under Chloe's skin, it's harder to face the reality of paying someone else to put our cat to death. At what point will we be certain that her suffering is greater than her pleasure? We are both beginning to regret our earlier, easily taken, platform on non-intervention, but we have passed the point of no return.

I can stay up all day without a nap, I report to Ed the surgeon. Just think, he replies, you used to take that for granted. Get a bilateral mammo in September, and come and see me in October.

Back to Irvine for a research fellowship and a search committee. The kid in the parking lot booth calls me sir. I give him ten dollars and get change without turning back into a madam.

Irvine again. Chungmoo wonders where I've been. On medical leave, I say. I have breast cancer. Pain on her face. Both her parents died of cancer.

I stop by to say hello to my old assistant. She doesn't recognize me. When she does she wants the hair back.

Alison from Cedars who kept me going by showing her fuzz is at the Hollywood farmers market. She doesn't recognize me. I don't stop her.

Anne calls in the evening, hysterical about the effects of surgery on her cat. Kim and I volunteer to go to the emergency animal hospital to get an Elizabethan collar. At least my cat doesn't have cancer, says the elderly woman in the deserted waiting room, apropos of nothing. They don't know what she has, but anything's better than cancer.

I tell my fellowship group that I will not be working on the Dominica book, as proposed, but on pulling together a manuscript about my year with breast cancer. I cannot get myself to think about the cultivation of limes and other colonial insanities. I cannot tear myself away from Her Baldness. It is, after all, a research group on autobiography. I glance at the group facilitators, whom I have already told, to ask permission to break the news, thinking, I suppose, that it would be bad form to throw the rock into the collegial banter. The news sinks without a ripple. *My wife had it,* Bob F. says to me afterwards, very quietly. *She's fine now.*

WEDNESDAY | APRIL 18, 2001

Reading of some of HB's missiles, as Yvonne calls them, at CalArts last night, with Matias and Leslie and Kaucyila. The event was part of a week arranged by the latest incarnation of a feminist art collective, the Toxic Titties, twenty-somethings all. *Oh,* I said, when they called to explain who they were and invited me, *no problem, that's perfect. I actually HAVE a toxic tittie.* I am certain such a possibility had never occurred to them. Leslie reads a piece that combines being bitten by a brown recluse with living in a Neutra house. I read BETH and the missile about chemo. The voice that describes the drip shakes. I can see people wince. No one actually wants to describe illness except people who have been there. No one grasps the nuances of the effort to pursue the body in degeneration except the people who have been there.

MONDAY | APRIL 23, 2001

Irvine. *How are you?* says the associate dean, whom I run into on my way out of a job candidate's slide lecture. *I MADE IT THROUGH!* I reply, doing a little jig in the courtyard. The associate dean thinks I am trashing the lecture. I have to backpedal. *No, I didn't mean that, the job candidate gave an absolutely wonderful talk. We'd be lucky to get him. I was on a medical leave this fall. Oh, that's right. You were off.*

TUESDAY | APRIL 24, 2001

I wouldn't do handstands in yoga, says Bob F. *You might get lymphedema. My wife did.*

SUNDAY | APRIL 29, 2001

Hollywood farmers market. *That woman was trying to talk to you,* said Kim. *She was bald and I told her you had had chemo but when she tried to get your attention you didn't see her.*

MONDAY | APRIL 30, 2001

You used to go into purgatory, said Kim. *I had to watch.* Nath sends a photograph. Her back is turned. She is standing on the stone wall at La Donine, throwing seeds and hair to the wind.

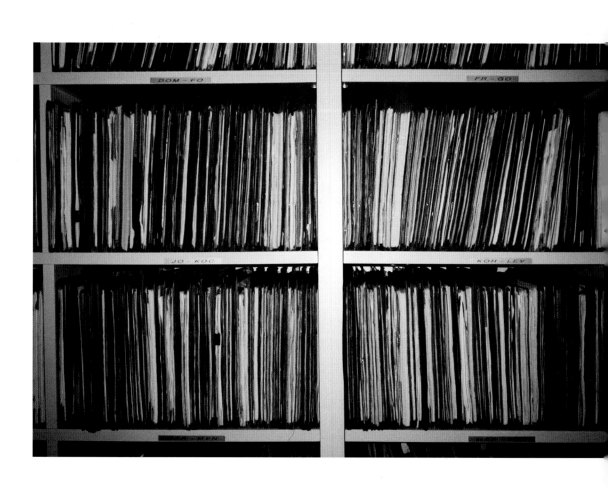

MAY | 2001

Reading at UCLA, again the saga of chemo and Jennifer's sculpture, this time for a panel on auto-biography. Neither an artist nor a toxic tittie in sight. Her Baldness props her laptop on the Sunset Garden book and reads from the screen. Lame as performance art, but HB feels the need to declare she is not a regular academic. Later, someone wonders whether she might be interested in doing something at a conference on disability. Feeling pretty good, getting back to being well, getting back into her real work, planning her trip to London for the summer, Her Baldness is stunned. The first, suspiciously vehement words out of my mouth: I'm not disabled.

Who says?

It's the new thing, it turns out, in the way of undoing normalcy. Maybe disability studies can out-run queer theory in the academic race for chic. Either I am a fraud—not as sick as others, not as impaired in my physical functioning—or I am in complete denial. What on earth do I suppose cancer is, if not a handicap?

FRIDAY | MAY 18, 2001

IN A MESSAGE DATED 5/18/01 CBLORD@UCI.EDU WRITES TO UNDISCLOSED RECIPIENTS:

SUBJECT: GERALDINE'S REFRIGERATOR

Her Baldness has been going back to her group, after more than a few months off. No matter how many cancer tests she passes with flying colors, she realizes that she is not finished with the company of her kind. There is wisdom to the structure that allows people with cancer to continue in support groups for eighteen months after the alleviation of their symptoms. Her Baldness was glad to find everyone she started with alive, though Suzie is very fragile. Suzie wept all night one night, she says, about being back to chemo again. On top of that she has to give herself a shot daily, one a day for two months, so that the pulmonary embolism she has developed will dissolve. It hurts. She isn't even halfway through her first box of syringes. Dotcom with the brain tumor wobbles when he stands, and his speech is slurred. He is careful to inform us that he comes only because his wife needs to be able to talk to the people in the group for family and friends in the next room.

Tom with pancreatic cancer is on a stronger recipe. His skin is dead white and his hair is thinner. He understands now, he says, what the ladies were talking about when they complained about chemo. He's softer, and this is not just a matter of muscle tone or the fatigue that makes him nod off on the sofa every now and again. He no longer leaps to lecture, although every now and then when someone else despairs, he pulls himself together and forcefully delivers his formula. You've got to set goals. I think of something I want to do in three weeks and I get there. I allow myself time to recuperate, and then I set another goal. I'm grateful for the time that I have.

Naomi has gotten cynical. She leaves work the minute she can in the afternoon, and if the traffic makes her late in the morning she doesn't mind. Glenda quit the group, went back to work, and sent word that she finished the Los Angeles marathon.

Doris the customs officer is also back on the job. The lines are awful, what with hoof and mouth disease. In the old days she would have jumped up and lent a hand whether or not her shift had started, but now she doesn't do a thing until she has to. She's glad she stopped carrying a gun because there are days she'd be happy to shorten the lines some other way. She's fixed up her porch just the way she always wanted but she doesn't go out there to sit. When she goes to the china store to add to her collections she can't make herself buy anything. She walks round and round the table of what used to be her favorite pattern until she wears a groove in the carpet but she cannot make a purchase.

Jane, a newcomer in her sixties, pancreatic cancer, feels awful with the chemo but tells her husband and family she feels just fine. She can't stand being cooked for, she can't stand them in her kitchen, and group is the only place where she can actually say she feels awful. Veronica, another newcomer, colon cancer, six rounds in all, two to go, is depressed. Prozac is not pulling her out. Her boyfriend dumped her when she started chemo. You don't want to be with him then, said Angela.

I'm sorry if it sounds like I'm giving you attitude but it's my esophageal cancer. It does something to my voice.

Have any of us felt like suicide? asks Veronica. Yes. She doesn't ask her friends for help because she doesn't want to wear them out. She doesn't ask the group for help because ours is a club to which she doesn't want to belong.

How are you? I am asked. When I say that I'm having trouble getting well, Greta is incredulous. She had a normal mammogram a year ago and now breast cancer has spread to her bones. She has just started chemo, she is exhausted, and she is mad at me because she cannot imagine I could or should be anything but grateful for my good fortune. I am out the other side. But I miss the intensity of illness. I miss the fear and I miss the adrenalin. I can now move in the world at full speed, and I am no longer afraid of being bumped or bruised by people who are moving more quickly than I, but they seem to me, almost always, thick and dull, brutish in their motions and often silly.

There is a membrane that separates the world of illness from the world of health and I am having trouble negotiating it. I can with no trouble at all slip into the world where I am not a breast cancer survivor unless I choose to be, unless I say something as a matter of ethics, or politics, unless I wear a pink ribbon, which I don't, unless I choose to make it an issue. It is not, however, the world that I always prefer. People no longer say that I look fabulous, they say that I look good. Though in general I decline to do so, I can pass. I can be a guy, or a white middle-aged female university professor with some sort of a tiresome affectation about her sexuality, or a woman who has been slashed and poisoned and burned and reemerged not at middle age but at the beginnings of old. My hair is entirely gray. My hands show age spots and my veins are ropy and the flesh underneath my chin sags. It doesn't matter that women tell me I look like a teenager or that my students say with relief, I was scared last spring when you got sick but now you look GREAT. Suddenly I can see myself, especially when caught in unfamiliar mirrors, in the body of my mother and of her mother: same thick hair, gray and wavy, same bulk in the shoulders and chest, same forward list.

What I am not obliged to be is a woman who had a bad mammogram exactly a year ago and who has four years to go before her chances of a recurrence decline to the point where she can take a deep breath because the offending breast will have achieved statistical normality. I can stand precisely at the edge of the membrane, so that if I tilt my head fractionally to one side I can see illness and if I tip my head to the other side I can see the world where people do not think of illness. Just as you can play under waterfalls that come off a smooth sheet of rock, moving from one side of the water to the other, standing inside and looking out to the sun, then standing outside and looking through to darkness and rock, I can move my body back and forth across the membrane and when I do I cannot help but smile because it is a delirium to be able to see both sides. You don't, however, if you can help it, want to stand there forever because the water gets heavy as it beats down on your head and shoulders and back. On one side of the line people don't know the membrane exists and on the other side of the line people cannot forget it exists.

It is now clear to Her Baldness that the mysterious presences and absences in her life during this past year were mainly but not entirely a result of knowledge or ignorance in respect to the existence of the membrane, rather than failings in her character or in the character of her friends. There are people she barely knew before her diagnosis who have been steady and hilarious presences, in spite of the chaos of their own lives. Her mother sent her a card every single week of her treatments, and her mother took care to thank the girlfriend for saving her daughter. Her brother-in-law sent her informative URLs every day. Her sister called every other day. Her Baldness has received astonishing phone calls, great gifts of time, and more smiley faces, cyber xxxxxxxs and LOLs than she could possibly count, not to mention chain letters invoking the Dalai Lama.

There are also people who vanished, only some of whom have resurfaced now that it is safe. There are close friends who failed her at crucial moments because they were so afraid of losing her that they had to go away. They were afraid of a hole in their lives and they could not be with their fear or with Her Baldness. For example, only recently did Her Baldness realize, after a long and painful talk with her friend Annie, that she would, in fact, have left an empty space in Annie's life, among others. Until that moment, she had interpreted the running as nothing other than selfishness.

When I first got my diagnosis, said Geraldine, I needed a new refrigerator but I didn't see the point of spending money so I went out and got a shitty one. In avocado. Here it is, six years later, and I'm still living with it. Her Baldness watches the newcomers arrive in her group while she waits for someone she knew at the beginning, when she joined, to die. She elicits from the newcomers, over and over again, descriptions of their fear, their depression, their denial, and their bargaining. She isn't proud of her behavior, but she had an experience that was too big for her the first time around and she needs to hit the rewind button. The only way to understand what it is that happened to her is to watch other people have what she had, which is, perhaps, why Geraldine feels the need to come back to group and speak to people who might otherwise make compromises about refrigerators.

TUESDAY | MAY 29, 2001

Chloe will not make it through the summer. I am going to London to work for two months. Kim and I have had the conversation. We will not put Chloe down before I leave. We do not want to shorten her life so that ours will be more convenient. Kim will have to decide when to kill Chloe and how to say goodbye. I am sparing myself the spectacle of what my own body might produce, and I am grateful to Kim for letting me. We do not say this directly to each other.

Her Baldness won't make it either. She will slip away to wait in the wings, just like the cancer that engendered her, though I hope there is never the opportunity for a curtain call and engendered is too simple a word for something that can pass through the holes that exist both on the street and on the net. It would be presumptuous to write HB's obituary, perhaps dangerous, but when I read back through these files it's clear that she began as a bad joke because she was the only way I could stand myself as a freak and that she couldn't stop the joke she had started because it kept her amused even if her readers weren't sure the joke was funny and didn't know how to put it to me that a lot of things beside hair were worth considering. It is also clear that if I'd lived the life I said I wanted—friends nearby, neighborhood and community, etc. etc., THAT fantasy—the space would have been so tight that I would have gotten battered by my own fear. Many of my friends don't live near me. My friends who live near me don't stay still. Her Baldness needed to net people so that I could stay in place.

Way back at the beginning, Susan S. said that cancer hadn't transformed her. It was just a cliché, she said. People just go back to who they were before they got sick. But now her photographs are huge, full of color and whirl and blur. They take up space.

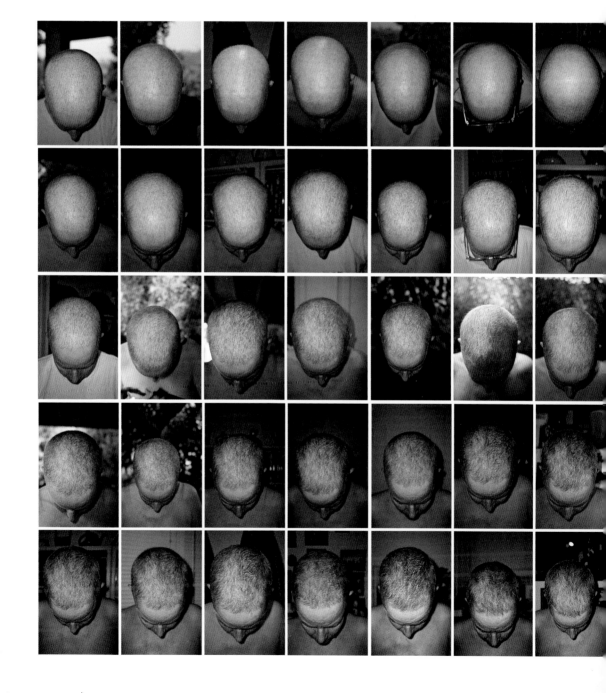

FEBRUARY | 2003

IN A MESSAGE DATED
2/14/03 CATHLORD WRITES
TO HER BALDNESS:

(A LETTER TO HER BALDNESS)

Dear H:

H is what I call you now, almost a year and a half after I thought I had seen you off to a good long hibernation. I don't remember where or when I lost the B. H stands for homo. H is hot. H is a way to avoid waves of nausea. H is Helen, the girl with blue eyes and black hair who was as unhappy as I was in boarding school. H is an homage to an undergraduate I have admired for some time, who achieved a limited celebrity by slashing his wrists in a performance art class when asked to use his body as material. (He got an incomplete, I think.) H is hero. Mostly, though, H is a way to tame you. It's easier to write dear H than it is to write dear HB, much less dear Her Baldness. I am not the sort of person who could be induced to correspond with an honorific. (Mrs. Honychurch confessed to me that she wouldn't buy a book with Her Baldness in the title because it made the author sound, well, rather self-important, and though I was hurt at the time, I see now what she meant.)

I need to talk. This is not to say that I miss you, because I can't decide whether I like you, but I am well aware that I owe you. You had no idea whether or not I would live, but you gave it your best shot. You were the pink triangle strategy: seize the negative stereotype, turn it around, use it proudly. Where on earth did you get the energy to write all those long emails? asked a friend. I was baffled by the question. You were my energy. You were all the energy I had.

Here's what's happened since we were last together.

One lump in my left breast, scheduled for biopsy on September 12, 2001. The biopsy was postponed for a week, allowing me to discuss American imperialism with Ed the surgeon while wearing a special visor—the breast center's latest boy toy, doubtless derived from military intelligence research—that made it possible for me to watch the image of his needle moving toward my lump. It turned out to be a cyst, a harmless thickening that under the circumstances felt absolutely trivial on the mortality scale. Otherwise, blood work every three months, extra mammo on the cancer side every six, and everything normal except for a bit of squamous on the driver's window side of my neck.

Kim's eighty-year-old father had to be unplugged after months of complications following open heart surgery. My almost-eighty-year-old mother caught colon cancer, made it through a resection, and declined chemo. A friend who was close long ago caught pancreatic cancer. Other friends caught the breast variety: Deb the photo historian, Dee Dee the tomato farmer whose mother died of breast cancer, Adrienne my graduate student, twenty-eight years old, who read an early passage from your rantings and went to the doctor to check on the hardness she had felt in her breast. Annetta had another mastectomy. She didn't tell me for months because she remembered she had promised to be a role model. Doris had a recurrence, more surgery and much more chemo. She is back at a desk job, in uniform but no gun. Let me also record the deaths: Marie Theophile's mother (cervical), Suzie (lung), Greta (breast), Julia Marie's sister-in-law (stomach), Jane (pancreatic) and Tom (ditto).

I have no problem calling Dr. Van Scoy Mosher by his first name.

I phone my mother as often as I can.

I am teaching. I invented a class on images of illness so that I could remind myself about fear in the presence of people who are too young to consider mortality on a regular basis. I like my students, and they like me. There are things we know we need to learn from each other. There are ideas it is my responsibility to teach. I am a calmer person. I pay closer attention.

Kim and I moved to a house that has room for both of us. In the process we renovated two kitchens and have not divorced. We argue about furniture and paint colors. We are not in agreement about whether or not to get a dog or adopt a child. I cannot as yet lay my hands on a book when I need it, and the wills I insisted we make vanished, along with the certificate for a free hair color job. We have two new cats, Sam and Lulu. I am planting an herb garden, into which I have dug Chloe's ashes, which I have kept ever since Kim put her down while I was in London celebrating my sister's fiftieth, the birthday she had to postpone because of my breast cancer. I am too busy to have gone to Macchu Picchu or the Alhambra or another silent retreat, but I have hiked to the oldest sequoia in California and to the pictographs in Horseshoe Canyon. I climbed Mont Sainte Victoire, Cezanne's mountain. I have not tackled Diablotin.

Joan Corbin and I have had tea, but the friends who made the donation that caused me to meet her have separated in bitterness.

No one has found a cure for cancer.

I look older and younger at the same time. People who ought to recognize me don't: e.g., old employers and famous white male artists on the elderly side. Like menopause, this gives me the delicious luxury of invisibility. I have begun taking anti-depressants because life is short and I don't want to waste it on depression.

I got a literary agent, a good New York one, who couldn't manage to sell you to a trade press. "People think there's definitely something there," she reported after a few months, "but no one can figure out the niche for your point of view." You're not marketable, H. On the other hand, I have been invited here and there to read some of your screeds. There is always a woman in the audience who wants to hear more. Translation: university press.

My voice comes from a place other than my body when I do these readings because it is hard, naturally, to revisit the place of my illness. It is much worse to sit in solitude and read you. Not only do you remind me of a time of fear and physical discomfort but you embarrass me. You spoke too loudly, as if speaking loudly and with all possible elegance would make valid the invalid. You spoke so loudly that often I couldn't hear what people were trying to say. (I didn't notice, for example, that one member of your list serv had developed a major crush on me.) You pontificated. You patronized. You were bossy. You were prone to rage. You were maudlin. Sometimes you cried at the keyboard. You were greedy. You snarled. You never admitted how lucky we were: a lover who stuck by us and never wavered in her generosity, friends, friends who are doctors, health insurance, tenure, generous medical leave, a garden to weed, getaways, restaurants, a computer, DSL. You were an overgrown, ungrateful, know-it-all, hormone-driven, vain, stuck-up teenager. You refused to be comforted. You rejected helpful suggestions out of hand. You did not understand that people were trying to tell you that they loved you. You used sarcasm to bury your dread. You were a compulsive joker. You tried too hard. You were a way to have things I didn't want to need because I thought they were clichés: cranio-sacral therapy, visions of vultures sitting on my chest, dreams, meditation, nutrition, etc.

Notwithstanding, you were way ahead of me. You recognized immediately that illness is a social space, a transparent bubble set down upon the person and her friends and her family and her colleagues and the strangers she encounters and the new people she meets. Illness is not something that happens to you but something you are — not someone's mother, for example, but the colon resection in room 235 that needs to be turned in the middle of the night. Illness is a transaction that involves other people, a lot of them. Illness is something in your body and of the air around your body. Being ill can make you sicker than cancer. Illness is lonely, all the more so because it affords you no solitude. The so-called private pain of illness is in fact an observed, calibrated, measured, unremittingly public space.

You mixed it up. You took what was private and made it public. You posted to the list serv emails intended to be personal. You published lists of gifts and their givers. You told tales on the support group, though of course you changed everyone's names. Conversely, you suppressed the sort of pathetic details that are the material from which pathographies are sculpted: explosive green diarrhea, prognosis, libido, state of caregiver's health, degree of depression, anger and envy of those who do not yet need to think about dying.

I discipline myself not to smooth away your unkindnesses as I engage in the fictions produced by the process of editing, combining, shuffling, arranging. I watch you turn from the being that kept me alive into a narrative device, a means to tell a story, a tool.

You fade.

When I try to rouse you by looking at photographs of my homely skinny bald self, I can remember neither the cadence of your speech nor the confusions of your accent. (In fairness, when I page through the books with lavender covers and the word BREAST in the title that I accumulated during the period of my medical interventions, I cannot remember a word of what I read.) It has taken me almost two years to understand that you are not the bald woman I see when I drag out the photographs from the summer of 2000. My baldness was the price I paid to know Her Baldness. I used you to spread my illness around other people's heads. I used you to make illness a space of language. You used words as bait. You trawled with your wit and your irony and your stubborn courage. I winched the net back to sort the catch.

I try to imagine whether I would want you back if and when my cancer returns. Would you be an old friend, or a mask for my shame? Would you have changed? Who would you be? Would I recognize you? Could I welcome you? Could I look forward to laughing at your gallows humor? Could I call you My Baldness, or will I need the third person? If I want you back, will you be there? Could I just BE sick, as Matias said way back when, rather than doing something about it? Would I by then MIND being bald?

It's not as simple as that.

I can't remember you because getting well is about forgetting, even though you are aware that you are losing something considerable in the forgetting. Being well is not an either/or thing. Getting well is a subtle process. You were not subtle.

I can't remember you because you disappeared gradually. You rewrote my understanding of friendship and frailty. In the process, my understanding of frailty and friendship wrote you out of existence.

I can't remember you because I replaced you. The list serv began as a device, a trick on my first bald evening, an abstraction to which I could send email. I needed abstraction at that moment. Do not underestimate the ugliness of skin so toxic that it kills what grows from it. Over time, you turned an abstraction into people. You caused the people I knew to sort themselves into another kind of family, a revised and enlarged nuclear family, the new and improved version of blood kin, the gene pool chiropractically adjusted so that responsibility is distributed all round amongst mothers and fathers and amusing uncles and children who never grew up and divas who left town and brothers who know how to do things and other brothers with a mean streak, not to mention platoons of unmarried women and boatloads of tomboys. This has been called the queer family, but the collectivity is much larger than that defined by sexual preference. Anyway, it's best to make a clean break with some relatives. Others are wonderful once every few years. Most can only provide certain things. Some can only take, and that, if you have something to spare, has its own pleasures.

Why it took me so long to see this will be another book.

That's not all. I can't remember you because when I had you I wanted to believe that cancer was a thing that came from outside of me. I could not admit that cancer was a thing that came from my body, a thing that erupted beneath my own skin, a thing inseparable from my body. I couldn't forgive myself. I had collaborated.

This is not the same as believing that the cancer was my fault.

So, H., I could go on like this—writing, reading, getting stuck in traffic jams, having conversations about art, making love, being late for faculty meetings, weeding, sharing meals with friends, taking the new cats to the vet, and, these days, going to demonstrations. Or, any day, without warning, I could be deported. There's no telling. I am aware of the suspense caused by an uncertainty, as I sit here writing, about whether or not I'll be here by the time this is published to give you the chance to read this. And if I am sent back, I may have to go it without you. But whether or not you're there, my crazy dented family will be. Whether or not I have the courage to go bald, I will get the courage by being bald. Bald is bigger than the absence of hair. J. G. Ballard, I remember reading, defines a prosthesis as the elevation of the castration complex to an art form. That could be the text for your wanted poster, H. Don't get literal about biology at this late stage. It's hard enough for a woman to use her head to make her way in the world, and it's harder when the hair on her own head betrays her.

C